This report contains the collective views of an international group of experts and does not necessarily represent the decisions or the stated policy of the United Nations Environment Programme, the International Labour Organisation, or the World Health Organization

Environmental Health Criteria 100

VINYLIDENE CHLORIDE

Published under the joint sponsorship of the United Nations Environment Programme, the International Labour Organisation, and the World Health Organization

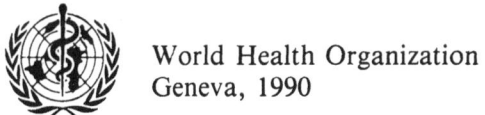

World Health Organization
Geneva, 1990

The International Programme on Chemical Safety (IPCS) is a joint venture of the United Nations Environment Programme, the International Labour Organisation, and the World Health Organization. The main objective of the IPCS is to carry out and disseminate evaluations of the effects of chemicals on human health and the quality of the environment. Supporting activities include the development of epidemiological, experimental laboratory, and risk-assessment methods that could produce internationally comparable results, and the development of manpower in the field of toxicology. Other activities carried out by the IPCS include the development of know-how for coping with chemical accidents, coordination of laboratory testing and epidemiological studies, and promotion of research on the mechanisms of the biological action of chemicals.

WHO Library Cataloguing in Publication Data

Vinylidene Chloride

(Environmental health criteria ; 100)

1.Vinylidene Chloride I.Series

ISBN 92 4 154300 0   (NLM Classification: QV 223)
ISSN 0250-863X

© World Health Organization 1990

Publications of the World Health Organization enjoy copyright protection in accordance with the provisions of Protocol 2 of the Universal Copyright Convention. For rights of reproduction or translation of WHO publications, in part or *in toto*, application should be made to the Office of Publications, World Health Organization, Geneva, Switzerland. The World Health Organization welcomes such applications.

The designations employed and the presentation of the material in this publication do not imply the expression of any opinion whatsoever on the part of the Secretariat of the World Health Organization concerning the legal status of any country, territory, city or area or of its authorities, or concerning the delimitation of its frontiers or boundaries.

The mention of specific companies or of certain manufacturers' products does not imply that they are endorsed or recommended by the World Health Organization in preference to others of a similar nature that are not mentioned. Errors and omissions excepted, the names of proprietary products are distinguished by initial capital letters.

Computer typesetting by HEADS, Oxford OX7 2NY, England

PRINTED IN FINLAND
Vammalan Kirjapaino Oy
DHSS — VAMMALA — 5500

CONTENTS

	Page
ENVIRONMENTAL HEALTH CRITERIA FOR VINYLIDENE CHLORIDE	10

1. SUMMARY AND CONCLUSIONS 11
   1.1 Properties, uses, and analytical methods 11
   1.2 Sources and levels of exposure 11
   1.3 Absorption, distribution, metabolism, and excretion 12
   1.4 Effects on experimental animals and cellular systems 12
       1.4.1 Covalent binding to tissues 12
       1.4.2 Acute toxicity 13
       1.4.3 Short-term studies 14
       1.4.4 Long-term studies 14
       1.4.5 Genotoxicity and carcinogenicity 15
       1.4.6 Reproductive toxicity 16
   1.5 Effects on human beings 16

2. IDENTITY, PHYSICAL AND CHEMICAL PROPERTIES, ANALYTICAL METHODS 17
   2.1 Identity 17
   2.2 Physical and chemical properties 19
   2.3 Analytical methods 21

3. SOURCES OF HUMAN AND ENVIRONMENTAL EXPOSURE 28
   3.1 Natural occurrence 28
   3.2 Production 28
   3.3 Uses 29
   3.4 Storage and transport 29

		Page
4.	ENVIRONMENTAL TRANSPORT, DISTRIBUTION, AND TRANSFORMATION	31

    4.1   Transport and distribution between media; degradation 31
           4.1.1   Air 31
           4.1.2   Water 32
           4.1.3   Soils and sediments 32
    4.2   Biodegradation 33
    4.3   Bioaccumulation 34

5. ENVIRONMENTAL LEVELS AND HUMAN EXPOSURE 35

    5.1   Air 35
           5.1.1   Ambient air 35
           5.1.2   Occupational exposure 36
    5.2   Water 37
    5.3   Soil 41
    5.4   Food and food packaging 42

6. KINETICS AND METABOLISM 45

    6.1   Animals 45
           6.1.1   Absorption 45
                    6.1.1.1   Inhalation exposure 45
                    6.1.1.2   Oral exposure 45
           6.1.2   Distribution and storage 46
           6.1.3   Elimination 46
                    6.1.3.1   Elimination of unchanged vinylidene chloride 47
                    6.1.3.2   Elimination of metabolites .. 48
           6.1.4   Metabolic transformation 50
           6.1.5   Reaction with cellular macromolecules 56
           6.1.6   Transformation by non-mammalian species 59
    6.2   Human beings 59

		Page

7. EFFECTS ON ORGANISMS IN THE
   ENVIRONMENT 61

   7.1 Effects on the stratospheric ozone layer 61
   7.2 Aquatic organisms 61

8. EFFECTS ON EXPERIMENTAL ANIMALS AND
   IN VITRO TEST SYSTEMS 63

   8.1 Single exposures 63
       8.1.1 Inhalation 63
             8.1.1.1 Rats 63
             8.1.1.2 Mice 71
             8.1.1.3 Other animal species 72
       8.1.2 Oral 73
             8.1.2.1 Rats 73
             8.1.2.2 Mice 78
       8.1.3 Other routes 78
             8.1.3.1 Intraperitoneal 78
             8.1.3.2 Eyes and skin 80
       8.1.4 Summary of acute toxicity 80
   8.2 Short-term exposures 80
       8.2.1 Inhalation 80
       8.2.2 Oral 84
   8.3 Long-term exposure 85
       8.3.1 Inhalation 85
       8.3.2 Oral 87
   8.4 Toxicity *in vitro* 89
   8.5 Mutagenicity and other genotoxicity assays ... 89
       8.5.1 Interaction with DNA 89
       8.5.2 Genotoxicity in bacteria 90
       8.5.3 Genotoxicity in yeast 93
       8.5.4 Genotoxicity in plants 94
       8.5.5 Genotoxicity in mammalian cells
             in vitro 94
       8.5.6 Genotoxicity in mammalian cells *in vivo* 95
       8.5.7 Summary 97
   8.6 Reproduction, embryotoxicity, and
       teratogenicity 104

		Page
8.7	Carcinogenicity	107
	8.7.1 Inhalation	107
	8.7.2 Oral	110
	8.7.3 Other routes	112
	8.7.4 Summary of carcinogenicity	113

9. EFFECTS ON HUMAN BEINGS 122

    9.1   Single and short-term exposures 122
    9.2   Long-term exposure 122

10. EVALUATION OF EFFECTS ON THE
ENVIRONMENT AND HUMAN HEALTH RISKS .. 126

    10.1   Evaluation of effects on the environment 126
    10.2   Evaluation of human health risks 126
              10.2.1 Levels of exposure 126
              10.2.2 Acute effects 127
              10.2.3 Long-term effects and genotoxicity ... 128

11. RECOMMENDATIONS 131

    11.1   Recommendations for future work 131
    11.2   Personal protection and treatment of poisoning 132
              11.2.1 Personal protection 132
              11.2.2 Treatment of poisoning in
                        human beings 133

12. PREVIOUS EVALUATIONS BY INTERNATIONAL
BODIES 134

REFERENCES 136

RESUME ET CONCLUSIONS, EVALUATION ET ....
    RECOMMANDATIONS 157

RESUMEN Y CONCLUSIONES, EVALUACION Y ...
    RECOMENDACIONES 173

WHO TASK GROUP ON VINYLIDENE CHLORIDE

Members

Dr M. Bignami, Laboratory of Ecotoxicology, Istituto Superiore di Sanita, Rome, Italy

Mr J.F. Howlett, Food Science Division, Ministry of Agriculture, Fisheries & Food, London, England (*Chairman*)

Professor C.L. Galli, Institute of Pharmacological Sciences, University of Milan, Milan, Italy

Professor E. Malizia, Emergency Toxicological Service, Antivenom Centre, Umberto the First Polyclinic, La Sapienza University, Rome, Italy

Dr K. Chipman, Department of Biochemistry, University of Birmingham, Birmingham, England

Dr Patricia S. Schwartz, Center for Food Safety and Applied Nutrition, Food & Drug Administration, Washington, DC, USA

Professor I.V. Sanotsky, Research Institute of Industrial Hygiene & Occupational Diseases, USSR Academy of Medical Sciences, Moscow, USSR (*Vice-Chairman*)

Dr R. Frentzel-Beyme, Institute for Documentation Information and Statistics, DKFZ, Heidelberg, Federal Republic of Germany (*Rapporteur*)

Dr J.F. Payne, Department of Fisheries and Oceans, St Johns, Newfoundland, Canada

Dr J.C. Parker, Office of Health & Environmental Assessment, US Environmental Protection Agency, Washington, DC, USA

Observers

Dr M.G. Penman, ICI Central Toxicology Laboratory, Macclesfield, Cheshire, England

Dr Chr. de Rooij, Solvay & Cie SA, Brussels, Belgium

Dr A. Mocchi, Centro Italiano Studi e Indagini (CISI), Rome, Italy

Secretariat

Mr J. Wilbourn, Unit of Carcinogen Identification and Evaluation, International Agency for Research on Cancer, Lyons, France

Dr E. Smith, International Programme on Chemical Safety, Division of Environmental Health, World Health Organization, Geneva, Switzerland (*Secretary*)

NOTE TO READERS OF THE CRITERIA DOCUMENTS

Every effort has been made to present information in the criteria documents as accurately as possible without unduly delaying their publication. In the interest of all users of the environmental health criteria documents, readers are kindly requested to communicate any errors that may have occurred to the Manager of the International Programme on Chemical Safety, World Health Organization, Geneva, Switzerland, in order that they may be included in corrigenda, which will appear in subsequent volumes.

* * *

A detailed data profile and a legal file can be obtained from the International Register of Potentially Toxic Chemicals, Palais des Nations, 1211 Geneva 10, Switzerland (Telephone no. 7988400/ 7985850).

ENVIRONMENTAL HEALTH CRITERIA FOR VINYLIDENE CHLORIDE

A WHO Task Group on Environmental Health Criteria for Vinylidene Chloride met in Rome, Italy, from 3 October to 7 October 1988. Dr E. Smith opened the meeting on behalf of the Director-General. The Task Group reviewed and revised the draft criteria document and made an evaluation of the health risks of exposure to vinylidene chloride.

The drafts of this document were prepared by Dr J.K. CHIPMAN, University of Birmingham, England. Dr E. SMITH, a member of the IPCS Central Unit, was responsible for the overall scientific content and Mrs M.O. HEAD, Oxford, England, for the editing.

The efforts of all who helped in the preparation and finalization of the document are gratefully acknowledged.

* * *

Financial support for the meeting was provided by the Ministry of the Environment of Italy; the Centro Italiano Studi e Indagini and the Istituto Superiore di Sanita, Rome, contributed to the organization and provision of meeting facilities.

Partial financial support for the publication of this criteria document was kindly provided by the United States Department of Health and Human Services, through a contract from the National Institute of Environmental Health Sciences, Research Triangle Park, North Carolina, USA – a WHO Collaborating Centre for Environmental Health Effects.

1. SUMMARY AND CONCLUSIONS

1.1 Properties, Uses, and Analytical Methods

Vinylidene chloride ($C_2H_2Cl_2$) is a volatile, colourless liquid with a "sweet" odour. It is stabilized with *p*-methoxyphenol to prevent the formation of explosive peroxides. Vinylidene chloride is used for the production of 1,1,1-trichloroethane and to form modacrylic fibres and copolymers (with vinyl chloride or acrylonitrile). Gas chromatographic methods have been developed for the determination of vinylidene chloride in air, water, packaging films, body tissues, food, and soil. The most sensitive method of detection is by electron capture.

1.2 Sources and Levels of Exposure

Up to approximately 5% of manufactured vinylidene chloride (representing an approximate maximum of 23 000 tonnes) is emitted into the atmosphere annually. The high vapour pressure and low water solubility favour relatively high concentrations in the atmosphere compared with those in other environmental "compartments". Vinylidene chloride in the atmosphere is expected to have a half-life of approximately 2 days.

Environmental levels in water are very low. Even in raw industrial waste water, the concentrations rarely exceed the µg/litre range, which is well below the mg/litre range of toxicity for aquatic organisms. The level in untreated drinking-water is generally not detectable. In treated, potable water, the levels of vinylidene chloride have generally been found to be < 1 µg/litre, though levels of up to 20 µg/litre have been detected. Levels of vinylidene chloride in food are usually not detectable, the maximum observed concentration being 10 µg/kg.

Occupational exposure to vinylidene chloride is mainly through inhalation, though skin or eye contamination can occur. Depending on the country, the maximum recommended or regulated time-weighted average (TWA) exposure limit is in the range of 8 to 500 mg/m^3, or else is the lowest reliably detectable concentration, depending on the country. Short-term exposure limits range from 16 to 80 mg/m^3 and ceiling values range from 50 to 700 mg/m^3.

1.3 Absorption, Distribution, Metabolism, and Excretion

Vinylidene chloride can be readily absorbed via the respiratory and oral routes in mammals, but data are not available on dermal absorption. Vinylidene chloride is widely distributed within the rodent body with concentrations reaching maximal levels in the liver and kidneys. The pulmonary elimination of unchanged vinylidene chloride is at least biphasic and dose dependent, being of greater importance at dose levels that saturate metabolism (approximately 600 mg/m^3 (150 ppm) via inhalation in the rat). Fasting of rats led to a reduction in the metabolism of an oral dose and a consequent higher level of exhaled vinylidene chloride.

The major routes of metabolism in the rat have been characterized. The predominant phase I metabolism involves cytochrome P-450 and the formation (possibly but not necessarily via an epoxide) of mono-chloroacetic acid. Cytochrome P-450 activity can be induced by vinylidene chloride. A number of phase I metabolites are conjugated with glutathione and/or with phosphatidyl ethanolamine prior to further conversions. Metabolism occurs at a greater rate in the mouse than in the rat resulting in a similar metabolic profile with a relatively higher proportion of glutathione conjugate derivatives. It has been shown that vinylidene chloride is also metabolized by human microsomal cytochrome P-450.

Metabolism of vinylidene chloride in rodents leads to depletion of glutathione and inhibition of the activity of glutathione-S-transferase.

1.4 Effects on Experimental Animals and Cellular Systems

1.4.1 Covalent binding to tissues

Covalent binding of [^{14}C]-vinylidene chloride-derived radiolabel occurs in the liver, kidney, and lung of rodents and is associated with toxicity in these organs. Covalent binding and toxicity are exacerbated by glutathione depletion and occur in the liver and

Summary and conclusions

kidney at a lower dose level in mice than in rats. A number of vinylidene chloride metabolites covalently bind to thiols *in vitro*.

1.4.2 Acute toxicity

Acute LC_{50} estimations for vinylidene chloride vary considerably, but this variation does not mask the fact that mice are much more susceptible to vinylidene chloride than rats or hamsters. Estimations of 4-h LC_{50} values ranged from approximately 8000 to 128 000 mg/m^3 (2000–32 000 ppm) in fed rats, 460–820 mg/m^3 (115–205 ppm) in fed mice, and 6640–11 780 mg/m^3 (1660–2945 ppm) in fed hamsters. Inaccuracies in LC_{50} estimations may arise because of a non-linear concentration-mortality relationship. Males of all species tended to have lower LC_{50} values than females, and fasting (which causes depletion of glutathione) increased toxicity in all three species. LD_{50} values following oral administration were approximately 1500 and 200 mg/kg in fed rats and mice, respectively. Acute inhalation toxicity in experimental animals was manifested as irritation of the mucous membranes, depression of the central nervous system, and progressive cardiotoxicity (sinus bradycardia and arrhythmias). Damage was caused to the liver, kidney, and lungs. In mice, which are more susceptible than rats to the hepatotoxicity and renal toxicity of vinylidene chloride, kidney damage and increased DNA replication were induced by exposure to as little as 40 mg vinylidene chloride/m^3 (10 ppm) for 6 h. As with inhalation, the principal organs affected by oral administration of vinylidene chloride are the liver, kidney, and lungs. The sequelae of events leading to hepatotoxicity appear to involve an early change in the bile canaliculi, which is followed by signs of mitochondrial damage. This precedes damage to the endoplasmic reticulum and cell death. Vinylidene chloride-induced liver and renal toxicity are apparently not caused by lipid peroxidation. Raised intracellular Ca^{++} concentrations may play a role in toxicity for the hepatocyte.

The toxic effects of vinylidene chloride are at least partially dependent on cytochrome P-450 activity (which may also be involved in detoxification) and can be exacerbated by glutathione depletion. Hepatotoxicity may be enhanced by ethanol and thyroxine, inhibited by dithiocarb and (+)-catechin, and modulated by acetone.

1.4.3 Short-term studies

Hepatic, renal, and, to a lesser extent, pulmonary damage have been observed in rodents exposed through inhalation to vinylidene chloride at 40–800 mg/m^3 for 4–8 h/day, 4 or more days/week, in short-term studies. Mice were more susceptible than rats, guinea-pigs, rabbits, dogs, and squirrel monkeys, and toxicity varied between different strains of mice. In general, female mice were less susceptible than males. Hepatotoxicity was reported in rats and mice exposed intermittently to vinylidene chloride concentrations of > 800 mg/m^3 (> 200 ppm) or 220 mg/m^3 (55 ppm), respectively. The levels required to produce hepatotoxicity through continuous exposure for several days were 240 mg/m^3 (60 ppm) for rats and 60 mg/m^3 (15 ppm) for mice. These intermittent and continuous treatments also caused nephrotoxicity in mice. The male Swiss mouse was particularly susceptible to vinylidene chloride-induced kidney toxicity. Male mice did not survive continuous short-term exposure to 200 mg vinylidene chloride/m^3 (50 ppm). The apparent no-observed-effect level for hepatotoxicity in dogs, squirrel monkeys, and rats was approximately 80 mg/m^3 (20 ppm) given as a continuous 90-day exposure. Short-term (approximately 3 months) oral dosing studies in rats (up to 20 mg/kg daily) and dogs (up to 25 mg/kg daily) did not show any evidence of toxicity other than minimal reversible hepatic damage in rats.

1.4.4 Long-term studies

Long-term studies of intermittent inhalation exposure to vinylidene chloride revealed that 300 mg/m^3 (75 ppm) caused only mild reversible hepatic changes in rats. At 600 mg/m^3 (150 ppm), the highest tolerable dose for long-term exposure in rats, liver damage with necrosis was evident. A high mortality rate with evidence of liver damage was observed in mice at 200 mg/m^3 (50 ppm). Kidney toxicity was evident following long-term treatment of mice at 100 mg/m^3 (25 ppm). Oral dosing of rats for one year with up to 30 mg vinylidene chloride/kg daily also produced minimal hepatic changes. These data do not provide a clear no-observed-effect

Summary and conclusions

level. There was some evidence from a separate study that renal inflammation and liver necrosis could be induced in rats and mice, respectively, following long-term oral administration of vinylidene chloride at daily dose levels of 5 mg/kg and 2 mg/kg, respectively.

1.4.5 Genotoxicity and carcinogenicity

Vinylidene chloride was found to be mutagenic for bacteria and yeast, only in the presence of a mammalian microsomal metabolic activation system (S9). The compound induced unscheduled DNA synthesis in isolated rat hepatocytes and increased the frequency of sister chromatid exchanges and chromosomal aberrations in cell cultures with S9 included. In contrast, no increase in mammalian gene mutations was seen. A small, but statistically significant, increase in DNA binding after *in vivo* exposure has been reported. DNA binding was greater in mouse than in rat cells and greater in the kidneys than in the liver following 6-h exposures to 40 and 200 mg vinylidene chloride/m^3 (10 and 50 ppm). Furthermore, vinylidene chloride slightly increased unscheduled DNA synthesis in mouse kidney. There was no evidence of a dominant lethal effect or cytogenetic effects after *in vivo* exposure of rodents, with the exception of one study showing the induction of chromosomal aberrations in the bone marrow of the Chinese hamster.

Carcinogenicity studies have been carried out on 3 animal species (rats, mice, and hamsters). In male Swiss mice, there was a clear indication of carcinogenicity (kidney adenocarcinoma) following long-term intermittent exposure to 100 or 200 mg vinylidene chloride/m^3 (25 or 50 ppm) but not to 0 or 40 mg/m^3 (0 or 10 ppm).

The kidney tumours may be related in some way to observed kidney cytotoxicity and it is possible that repeated kidney damage either leads directly to the carcinogenic response by a non-genotoxic mechanism or facilitates the expression of the genotoxic potential of metabolites in this particular species, sex, and organ. However, this conclusion is uncertain in the light of the limited available data on genetic effects *in vivo* and the findings that vinylidene chloride may have acted as an initiator.

In the same study, statistically increased incidences of lung tumours (mainly adenomas in mice of both sexes) and mammary carcinomas (in females) were observed, but no dose-response relationships were found. In adult rats exposed through inhalation, a slight non-dose-related increase in mammary tumours was reported as well as a slight increase in leukaemia when rats were exposed *in utero* and then postnatally. These observations could not be evaluated.

1.4.6 Reproductive toxicity

No evidence was found of effects on fertility in rats continuously exposed to vinylidene chloride (up to 200 mg/litre, 200 ppm) in drinking-water. Inhalation of up to 1200 mg vinylidene chloride/m^3 (300 ppm), for 22–23 h, by rats and mice during various periods of organogenesis did not induce fetal abnormalities, other than those attributable to maternal toxicity.

Inhalation of up to 640 mg vinylidene chloride/m^3 (160 ppm) for 7 h/day in rats and rabbits or oral intake of approximately 40 mg/kg per day in rats during critical periods of gestation did not have any effects on embryos or fetuses at a level below that which produced maternal toxicity, but embryo and fetal toxicity and fetal abnormalities were seen at levels producing maternal toxicity, as evidenced by decreased weight gain.

1.5 Effects on Human Beings

Concentrations of vinylidene chloride of 16 000 mg/m^3 (4000 ppm) cause intoxication that may lead to unconsciousness. Stabilized vinylidene chloride is also an irritant for the respiratory tract, eyes, and skin. Kidney and liver damage have been reported for sub-anaesthetic, prolonged or repeated short-term exposures. Evaluation of epidemiological studies was hampered by limited cohort sizes, co-exposure to vinyl chloride, and insufficient attention to smoking habits. No statistically significant increased incidence of cancer was found in human beings exposed to vinylidene chloride, but the epidemiological studies were inadequate and it is not possible to conclude that there is no carcinogenic risk. No information is available on the effects of vinylidene chloride on reproduction in human beings.

2. IDENTITY, PHYSICAL AND CHEMICAL PROPERTIES, ANALYTICAL METHODS

2.1 Identity

Vinylidene chloride is a halogenated aliphatic hydrocarbon.

Chemical structure:

$$\begin{array}{c c} Cl & H \\ | & | \\ C & = C \\ | & | \\ Cl & H \end{array}$$

Molecular formula: $C_2H_2Cl_2$

Relative molecular mass: 96.95

Common synonyms: 1,1-dichloroethylene; 1,1-dichloroethene; 1,1-dichloro; VDC; 1,1-DCE; VC; vinylidene dichloride; chlorure de vinylidene (France); asym-dichloroethylene; NCI-C54262

Common trade name: Sconatex

IUPAC systematic name: 1,1-dichloroethylene

NCI number: C54262

CAS registry number: 75-35-4

RTECS number: KV9275000

EEC number: 602-025-00-8

Conversion factors:
1 ppm vinylidene chloride = 4 mg/m^3
1 mg vinylidene chloride/m^3 = 0.25 ppm
at 25 °C, 1 atm.

Commercial vinylidene chloride

The technical product (which is >99.6% pure) can contain impurities (Table 1).

Table 1. Maximum levels of impurities found in commercial vinylidene chloride[a]

Dichloroacetylene	10 mg/kg
Monochloroacetylene	1 mg/kg
Vinyl chloride	20 mg/kg
Water	100 mg/kg
Acidity (as HCL)	15 mg/kg
Iron	0.5 mg/kg
Peroxides (as H_2O_2)	1 mg/kg
Other halogenated impurities	500 mg/kg (total)

[a] From: ECETOC [45].

Note: Hydroquinone monomethyl ether (*p*-methoxyphenol) is the most commonly used inhibitor, which is added at a level of 50–200 mg/kg. The carcinogen dichloroacetylene may also occur as an impurity, as it is a by-product of vinylidene chloride synthesis [185].

2.2 Physical and Chemical Properties

The principal physical and chemical properties of vinylidene chloride are shown in Table 2.

Table 2. Some physical and chemical properties of vinylidene chloride[a]

Physical form	volatile, clear, colourless liquid; it polymerizes readily in the presence of oxygen above 0 °C
Odour	"sweet" odour; apparent detection limit for human beings, approximately 2000–4000 mg/m$_3$ [b]
Boiling point (°C)	31.56
Freezing point (°C)	−122.5
Relative density (20 °C/40 °C)	1.213
Vapour density (air = 1, 20 °C)	3.34
Density in saturated air (air = 1)	2.8
Vapour pressure (mmHg) at:	
−20 °C	7
0 °C	215
20 °C	495
25 °C	591
Refractive index (N_D) (20 °C)	1.4247
Viscosity (P·s) (20 °C)	0.3302
Critical temperature (°C)	220.8
Critical pressure (atm)	51.3
Heat of combustion (kcal/mol) (25 °C)	261.9 (liquid monomer)

Table 2 (contd).

Heat of formation (kcal/g)	−25.1 (liquid monomer) 1.26 (gaseous monomer)
Solubility in water (21 °C)	2.5 g/kg
Solubility in organic solvents:	very soluble – diethyl ether, chloroform soluble – benzene, acetone, ethanol
Calculated log n-octanol/water partition coefficient	1.66[c]
Flash point (open cup) (closed cup)	-15 °C -19 °C
Flammability limits in air (% vol)	5.6–16
Saturation concentration in air (20 °C)	2640 g/m^3
Autoignition temperature (°C)	513
Heat of evaporation (31.6 °C) (cal/mol)	6.3
Heat of polymerization (25 °C) (kcal/mol)	18

[a] From: Buckingham [22], Gibbs & Wessling [59], Hushon & Kornreich [84], Shelton et al. [201], Weast [241], and Wessling & Edwards [243], unless stated otherwise.
[b] From: Torkelson & Rowe [222].
[c] From: Rekker [187].

In the absence of a stabilizer and in the presence of oxygen, vinylidene chloride forms an explosive peroxide at temperatures as low as −40 °C [22]. The decomposition products of vinylidene chloride peroxides include phosgene, formaldehyde, and hydrochloric acid [59]. Vinylidene chloride also reacts vigorously with oxidizing materials and is highly dangerous when exposed to heat or flame [197]. It undergoes addition reactions as in the formation of 1,1,1-trichloroethane when it is reacted with hydrogen chloride. Alcohols and halides react with vinylidene chloride to give carboxylic acids [22]. Vinylidene chloride will react with aluminium to form reactive aluminium chloroalkyls, and copper can form reactive acetylides from its interaction with acetylenic impurities. In the presence of a polymerization initiator, vinylidene chloride forms homopolymers and copolymers with other vinyl monomers [59].

2.3 Analytical Methods

Some spectral features of vinylidene chloride are shown in Table 3. Vinylidene chloride is well suited to liquid and headspace sampling and determination by gas chromatography. Details of sampling, preparation, and the determination of vinylidene chloride in different media are given in Table 4. The major analytical limitation is interference by other constituents of the media.

Table 3. Ultraviolet absorption and mass spectroscopic characteristics of vinylidene chloride

UV absorption maximum	200 vap[a]		
Mass spectrum	61 (100)	96 (61)[b]	
	98 (38)	63 (32)	
	26 (16)	60 (15)	
	25 (7)	35 (6)	

[a] From: Weast [241].
[b] From: Grasselli & Ritchey [63].

Table 4. Sampling, preparation, and determination of vinylidene chloride[a]

Medium	Sampling method	Analytical method[b]	Detection limit	Comments	Reference
Air	Cold trap (liquid O_2) using column of glass beads; desorb thermally by purge			Introduction of a sorbent trap allows a large sample; however, cumbersome for handling	[212]
	Trap with pyridine in cooled impinger	Colourimetric measurement of derivative (cyanine)	10 mg/m^3		[66]
	Trap with charcoal; desorb with CS_2	GC/FID	1 µg/m^3 (7 µg/sample tube)	Well suited for monitoring occupational exposure levels; trapped vinylidene chloride is stable for at least 16 days; when desorbed in CS_2, analysis should be within 4 days; humidity dramatically reduces the breakthrough volume	[50] [205] [80]
	Trap with adsorbent column; desorb thermally	GC/FID	4 µg/m^3		[191] (see also [199])
	Trap with charcoal desorb with CS_2	GC/FID	working range 2–20 mg/m^3 for a 5- to 7-litre sample		[226]

Table 4 (contd).

Human breath	Trap with Tenax polymer; desorb thermally	GC/MS	0.12 µg/m³ (0.6 µg/m³, quantifiable limit)	Suitable for monitoring environmental samples [233]
Human breath	Spirometer used for sampling; trap and desorb as above	GC/MS	0.16 µg/m³ (0.82 µg/m³, quantifiable limit)	[233]
Human breath	As above using liquid nitrogen cryogenic trap	GC/MS	0.16 µg/m³ (0.82 µg/m³, quantifiable limit)	[233, 234]
Vinyl chloride	Distillates	GC/FID	5 mg/kg	[107]
Water[c]	Direct injection	Steam-modified G-solid C/FID	approx. 5 µg/litre	Obvious advantages of direct injection but rapid deterioration of column [67]
	Direct headspace analysis (purge and trap between water columns)	GC/FID confirmation by MS	2 µg/litre	[171]
	Dynamic headspace technique	(a) GC/FID (b) GC/ECD	(a) 0.5 µg/litre (b) 0.1 µg/litre	[162]

Table 4 (contd).

Medium	Sampling method	Analytical method[b]	Detection limit	Comments	Reference
Water (contd)	Static headspace technique	GC/FID	5 µg/litre (quantifiable limit)		[164]
		GC/ECD	10 µg/litre (quantifiable limit)		
	Purge with inert gas; trap (Tenax); desorb as vapour	GC/ECD	0.13 µg/litre	A microcoulometric detector can also be used; direct aqueous injection above 0.13 mg/litre	[223]
		GC/FID and EC	1 µg/litre	Linearity shown for response versus concentration between 10 µg/litre and 1 mg/litre[d]	[17] [234]
	As above with isotope-labelled vinylidene chloride as internal standard	GC/MS	10 µg/litre	Internal standard corrects for variability in recovery	[224]
	Headspace transfer (vacuum distillation) to cryogenic trap	GC/EC	0.03 µg/litre	Sensitive and inexpensive – recommended for field conditions	[31]

Table 4 (contd).

	Purge-closed loop method	GC/EC, EDC, or FID (most efficient not indicated)	0.2 µg/litre (20-ml sample)	Combines gas-stripping and static headspace methods - recommended as an effective, reliable and rapid method for routine sample analysis	[236]
Packaging materials (Saran films)	Films dissolved in tetrahydrofuran or carbon tetrachloride; can be injected with solvent-flush technique	G-solid C/EC confirmation by MS	5 mg/kg	Injection port needs cleaning regularly	[18]
			1 mg/kg		[78]
		GC/MS	1 mg/kg		[144, 218]
	Vinylidene chloride released thermally; sample by headspace technique	GC/FID		Requires internal standard of polymer with known content of vinylidene chloride	[62]
	Headspace technique	GC/EC	1 µg/m²		[60]
Food simulating solvents exposed to Saran films (corn oil, heptane, and water)	Headspace technique	G-solid C/EC confirmation by MS	5–20 µg/kg		[78]
		GC/EC	1 µg/kg		[238]

Table 4 (contd).

Medium	Sampling method	Analytical method[b]	Detection limit	Comments	Reference
Food	Headspace technique	GC/EC	5 µg/kg		[60]
Body tissues (various)	Minced tissue added to iso-octane/water; purge (helium); trap (Tenax); desorb as vapour	GC/ECD	approximately 10 µg/kg (limit of detection of injected material, 50 pg)	Well suited for pharmacokinetic studies; specific purging method avoids foaming	[125]
Body tissue (fish)	Tissue homogenized; purge and trap procedure	GC/MS	10 µg/kg	Recovery reported better by vacuum distillation method	[44] [76]
Soil	Extract (n-hexadecane); add internal standard	GC/EC	10 µg/kg		[37]
Sediment	Sealed in vial with internal standard; purge with inert gas; trap (Tenax); desorb	GC/EC	5 µg/kg	Minimum recovery observed = 67%	[214]

a Methods for grab sampling of air are not included, since these do not allow estimations of time-weighted average values; laser Stark spectroscopy [215] or portable infrared analysers [50] give poor sensitivity and specificity due to interference by other halohydrocarbons.

b GC = gas chromatography;
   FID = flame ionization detection;
   EC = electron capture;
   EDC = electrolytic conductivity;
   MS = mass spectroscopy.

c If the sample contains chlorine, sodium thiosulfate should be added to prevent chlorination of hydrocarbons [17].
d From: Ramstad et al.[181].

3. SOURCES OF HUMAN AND ENVIRONMENTAL EXPOSURE

3.1 Natural Occurrence

Vinylidene chloride is not known to occur naturally.

3.2 Production

Crude vinylidene chloride is produced by the treatment of 1,1,2-trichloroethane with sodium hydroxide or calcium hydroxide. Fractional distillation of the washed and dried crude product provides the commercial vinylidene chloride to which a stabilizer (usually p-methoxyphenol) is added to prevent polymerization [59, 201].

Vinylidene chloride has also been shown to be produced in substantial quantities from the thermal decomposition of methyl chloroform [61]. Methyl chloroform vapours (1910 mg/m^3) decomposed to vinylidene chloride at temperatures above 350 °C and 180 °C in the absence and presence of copper, respectively. The extent to which this dehydrohalogenation occurs in work environments leading to human exposure to vinylidene chloride is not known. It has been demonstrated [220] that 1,1,1,2-tetrachloroethane is readily converted to vinylidene chloride *in vivo* in the rat by reductive metabolism. Thus, 1,1,1,2-tetrachloroethane is a potential source of bioavailable vinylidene chloride. In addition, vinylidene chloride is a major aqueous abiotic degradation product of a frequent contaminant of ground water, namely 1,1,1-trichloroethane [169, 230].

In 1967, world production of vinylidene chloride was estimated at 220 000–330 000 tonnes [201]. The following annual world production rates of vinylidene chloride (in thousands of tonnes) have been reported for the early 1980s [86]: the Federal Republic of Germany, 100; France, 50; Japan, 23; the Netherlands, 12; the United Kingdom, 30; and the USA, 90.7. This totals 306 000 tonnes. The estimates should be taken as very approximate and it is likely that the production level has now decreased [86]. A recent estimate of worldwide production is 290 000 tonnes annually: in Western Europe, approximately 80% of the vinylidene chloride produced is for internal use by the companies concerned (personal communication: European Chemical Industry Ecology and Toxicology Centre).

3.3 Uses

Vinylidene chloride is used for the production of 1,1,1-trichloroethane and to form modacrylic fibres and copolymers (Saran®) with alkyl acrylates, methacrylates, acrylonitrile, vinyl acetate, or vinyl chloride [59]. Vinylidene chloride/vinyl chloride copolymers (Saran® B) are used for the packaging of foods, as metal coatings in storage tanks, building structures, and tapes, and as moulded filters, valves, and pipe fittings. These copolymers are also used to reinforce polyesters, inks, and composites for furniture upholstery and other constructions. Polyvinylidene chloride or vinylidene chloride copolymerized with acrylic esters or with acrylonitrile and acrylic esters (Diofane®) are used for coating paper and board and as flame-retardant binders in other coatings. It is prohibited in the EEC to include vinylidene chloride in cosmetics [88]. Regulations in the USA [88] restrict the vapour concentration of vinylidene chloride to 25% of the lower explosive limit when used in spray finishing operations.

3.4 Storage and Transport

The storage and transport of vinylidene chloride may be sources of exposure; however, reports of such exposure have not been found in the literature. Vinylidene chloride should not be stored for more than a day without a stabilizer [59], which does not need to be removed prior to use in polymer syntheses. The monomer should be blanketed with inert gas, stored (e.g., hermetically sealed steel containers) at a maximum of $-10\,^\circ$C and protected from light, air, free radical initiators, copper, and aluminium [201] (section 2.2). Under these conditions, inhibited vinylidene chloride can be transported and stored, though the length of the storage period should be minimal. A water-spray system should be available for cooling the tanks in the event of fire. Containers of vinylidene chloride must be appropriately labelled. In the EEC, the following labels apply: extremely flammable, harmful by inhalation, possible risk of irreversible effects, keep container tightly closed, keep away from sources of ignition, no smoking, do not empty into drains [88]. Any industrial waste containing this substance must be listed as hazardous and is therefore subject to handling, transport, treatment, storage, and disposal regulation. Disposal should be by incineration and not by discharge into sewers. Complete combustion should be ensured to prevent the formation of phosgene. An acid scrubber should be used to remove the halo-acids produced. Vinylidene chloride-derived peroxides can be detected by the liberation of iodine following the addition of acidified isopropanol saturated with sodium iodide and can be destroyed by contact with water at room temperature [201].

4. ENVIRONMENTAL TRANSPORT, DISTRIBUTION, AND TRANSFORMATION

4.1 Transport and Distribution Between Media, Degradation

4.1.1 Air

The high vapour pressure and low water solubility of vinylidene chloride favour relatively high atmospheric concentrations compared with other environmental "compartments". Atmospheric radicals will play a major role in the degradation of vinylidene chloride. The rate constant for oxidation of vinylidene chloride with hydroxyl radicals (the major reacting radical) was reported to be 4×10^{-12} cm^3/mol per second [34]. Judging by this and the half-lives of related chlorinated ethenes reacting with hydroxy radicals, the half-life of vinylidene chloride reacting with tropospheric hydroxyl radicals (assumed to be 10^{-6} radicals/cm^3) is expected to be approximately 2 days. Degradation by reaction with other atmospheric radicals will also take place. Vinylidene chloride may react with chlorine atoms derived from chloro-olefins, peroxy radicals (estimated half-life for this reaction in the atmosphere is 22 years; [20] and ozone (estimated half-life is 219 days; [225]. The gas-phase ozonolysis of vinylidene chloride at 25 °C follows second-order kinetics and appears to involve a chain mechanism the chain carrier being C Cl$_2$O. The products of the reaction are C Cl$_2$O, HCOOH, CH$_2$ClCCl(O), CO, O$_2$, HCl, and H$_2$O [83]. The chloroacetyl chloride is most likely formed by a rearrangement of 1,1-dichloroethylene oxide [58]. The measured half-life of vinylidene chloride within sealed quartz flasks exposed outdoors in the northwest of England [169] was higher than expected from the information given above (56 days). However, the relevance of these data to the environmental persistence of vinylidene chloride is difficult to interpret considering the high concentration used (80 mg/m^3) and the specific conditions of exposure.

The very long half-lives estimated for removal by rain droplets (1.1×10^5 years) or by adsorption on aerosol particles (1.5×10^8 years) indicates that these processes are insignificant [34].

4.1.2 Water

Consideration of the physical and chemical properties of vinylidene chloride (section 2.2) suggests that volatilization is the major transport process from water [46]. Dilling [40] measured the half-life for the evaporation of vinylidene chloride (1 mg/ml) from a stirred aqueous solution at 25 °C and with a depth of 6.5 cm. The value obtained (27.2 min) was remarkably close to the calculated value (20.1 min). Using the calculated re-aeration rate constant for vinylidene chloride and oxygen [127], a half-life can be calculated of between approximately 6 days (static pond water) and approximately 1 day (mobile river water).

Photolysis and hydrolysis are not likely to be significant [127], though degradation of vinylidene chloride in water contained in sealed bottles in the dark was apparently measurable (albeit slow) in the study by Pearson & McConnell [169]. The dispersal of vinylidene chloride was monitored by Wang et al. [236] following its discharge and mixing into a drainage canal that led to a river 1.5 km downstream. The maximum discharge water concentration of vinylidene chloride was 36.7 µg/litre. Midway canal water concentrations of vinylidene chloride were not only dependent on the concentration in the discharged water but were also inversely related to the canal flow rate. The highest midway canal water concentration was 1.4 µg/litre, which arose from a discharged concentration of 16.7 µg/litre with a canal flow rate of about 200 litres/second. At the site of confluence of the canal and river, the levels of vinylidene chloride were consistently less than 0.2 µg/litre (detection limit).

4.1.3 Soils and sediments

Few data are available on the transport or persistence of vinylidene chloride in soils and sediments.

The transformation of vinylidene chloride was studied in anoxic microcosms containing organic sediment collected from the Everglades in Southern Florida [13]. The first order rate constant of dehalogenation was 3.57×10^{-4} h^{-1} for surficial sediment and 1.67×10^{-4} h^{-1} for bottom sediments. Transformation products included low levels of vinylidene chloride but mechanisms of transformation other than reductive dechlorination occurred. The log n-octanol/water partition coefficient of 1.66 [187] and the significant solubility of vinylidene chloride in water (2.5 g/litre) suggest that some leaching from soils may occur. As with water, volatilization is expected to be a major process of removal.

Relatively high concentrations of vinylidene chloride (1600 ± 400 µg/litre) have been reported in municipal wastewaters (primary treatment waters) in Orange Country, California [246]. However, quantifiable concentrations of vinylidene chloride (> 5 µg/kg) were not found in sediments in the outfall area.

4.2 Biodegradation

Tabak et al. [217] measured a microbial degradation of 78% of vinylidene chloride (5 mg/litre) following 7 days incubation at 25 °C in a static culture flask, in the dark, with settled domestic waste water as microbial inoculum. With subsequent incubations (after adaptation), 100% loss of compound occurred. At 10 mg vinylidene chloride/litre, 45% loss was found in the first 7 days incubation. Volatilization losses over 7 days at 25 °C were 24 and 15% at 5 and 10 mg/litre, respectively. Activated sludge treatment of waste water resulted in 97% removal of vinylidene chloride at an inflow concentration of 0.04 mg/litre [168]. These data suggest a possible role of biodegradation; however, the evidence is not conclusive and volatilization may be responsible for some of the measured losses from the hydrosphere (inadvertent in the former study).

Recently, a mixed culture of methane-utilizing bacteria was found to degrade vinylidene chloride from 630 to 200 µg/litre following incubation in sealed culture bottles for 48 h. The products were non-volatile chlorinated substances and the corresponding amount of degradation using a dead culture was from 520 to 350 µg/litre [51]. Vogel & McCarty [230] have reported that anaerobic microorganisms can completely convert vinylidene chloride to vinyl chloride by reductive dehalogenation. Vinyl chloride can subsequently be mineralized to carbon dioxide.

4.3 Bioaccumulation

Bioaccumulation is expected to be low, based on the n-octanol/water partition coefficient and the water solubility (Table 2). A bioconcentration factor of 4 and a bioaccumulation factor of 6.9 were reported for fish in a review by Atri [9].

5. ENVIRONMENTAL LEVELS AND HUMAN EXPOSURE

5.1 Air

5.1.1 Ambient air

In an assessment of vinylidene chloride emission in the USA [84], an annual release of a total of 599 tonnes was estimated from production and polymerization operations. A more recent estimate of this emission is placed at a much lower level of 93.5 tonnes (personal communication, US Chemical Manufacturers Association, 1987). It was estimated that between 2 and 5% of vinylidene chloride manufactured in the USA was emitted into the air (20–50 tonnes per 1000 tonnes produced) [212] but, on the basis of current experience, the emissions into the air are of the order of 1%. With an annual global production of around 300 000 tonnes, the total emissions would be 3000 tonnes per year (personal communication, European Chemical Industry Ecology and Toxicology Centre).

Vinylidene chloride levels detected in ambient air from a petrochemical manufacturing area and a non-industrial centre, respectively, ranged from 0.06 to 416.07 $\mu g/m^3$ (mean, 46.84 $\mu g/m^3$) and from 3.53 to 27.29 $\mu g/m^3$ (mean, 11.21 $\mu g/m^3$) [233]. There was, therefore, marked variability. The concentrations in the breath of human individuals in the respective areas were in the ranges of 0.08–25.17 $\mu g/m^3$ and 3.94–14.12 $\mu g/m^3$. The data suggested a log-linear relationship between air and breath concentrations of vinylidene chloride (section 6.2). Hushon & Kornreich [84] reported the results of a US EPA ambient air sampling programme. Concentrations of vinylidene chloride ranged from not detectable to a maximum of 0.010 mg/m^3. In the rural northwest of the USA, in the mid 1970s [65], vinylidene chloride levels in air were non-detectable (< 20 ng/m^3; < 5 ppt), which is in accordance with the short half-life estimated for vinylidene chloride in the atmosphere (section 4.1.1). At the perimeters of industrial sites in the USA, air levels ranged from non-detectable up to 52 $\mu g/m^3$ [62] 0.6 miles from the site being the maximum distance for the detection of vinylidene chloride. In urban environments in the USA, mean air concentrations were found to be 19.6, 50.4, and 119.2 ng/m^3 (4.9, 12.6, and 29.8 ppt) [212]. These authors estimated average daily doses of 0.4, 1.1, and 2.5 µg/day, respectively, at these sites, based on a total air intake of 23 m^3/day. In a subsequent study [213] of seven additional cities in the USA, concentrations ranged from below the detection limit (20 ng/m^3; 5 ppt) to 0.224 µg/m^3, with arithmetic averages ranging from 0 to 0.123 µg/m^3. The median concentration of vinylidene chloride in the seven cities was 0.036 µg/m^3. Wallace et al. [235] reported a 5-year US EPA study in urban populations of personal exposures to vinylidene chloride amongst many other pollutants. A total of nearly 5000 air, breath, and drinking-water samples were collected for 400 respondents in New Jersey, North Carolina, and North Dakota. The median coefficients of variance for the analysis of air and breath samples was 20–40%. Vinylidene chloride was quantifiable, exceeding approximately 1 µg/m^3 only occasionally (<10% measurable).

Vinylidene chloride concentrations in the 1.640–4.08 µg/m^3 (0.35–1.02 ppb) range were measured at urban sites in New Jersey as part of the Airborne Trace Element and Organic Substances (ATEOS) project [68, 69]. However, the authors considered that the relatively high concentrations of vinylidene chloride found may be an artifact of 1,1,1–trichloroethane dehydrochlorination on the particular adsorption traps (Tenax GC) used in the study. US EPA [225] estimated the ambient airborne level of vinylidene chloride to be 8.7 µg/m^3 and 20 ng/m^3 in industrial-source and non-industrial areas of the USA, respectively. In the Federal Republic of Germany, vinylidene chloride is classed among a group of organic compounds, the total emission of which must not exceed a concentration of 20 mg/m^3 at a mass flow of 0.1 kg/h or more [88].

5.1.2 Occupational exposure

Industrial air concentrations of vinylidene chloride should be restricted. Ott et al. [166] reported peak air exposure levels as high as 7600 mg/m^3 in a polymer production plant with operators being exposed to estimated 8-h time-weighted average (TWA) concentrations of between <20 and 280 mg/m^3. In a more recent survey in the USA [225], levels of vinylidene chloride in monomer and polymer plants were reported of 90–100 µg/m^3 and 25–50 µg/m^3, respectively. Thus, exposures are generally within the time-weighted average threshold limit value (TLVR) of 20 mg/m^3 (5 ppm), recommended by the ACGIH (Table 5). Similarly, vinylidene chloride levels in air in other manufacturing plants [91, 111,165] where exposure to vinylidene chloride was involved have been reported to be below 40 mg/m^3. This was also the case for occupational exposures in confined atmospheres (submarines and spacecraft) [1] and in certain USA telephone offices [155] where the airborne levels of vinylidene chloride were found not to exceed 8 mg/m^3 and 256 µg/m^3, respectively.

Some national occupational exposure limits are listed in Table 5.

5.2 Water

Vinylidene chloride has been measured in raw and treated effluents discharged from various industrial plants in the USA [225]. The mean levels detected in raw waste water in the USA ranged from 18 to 760 µg/litre. Vinylidene chloride (isomer not specified) has been detected in effluent discharged from chemical manufacturing plants in the Netherlands at a concentration of 32 µg/litre [47]. Going & Spigarelli [62] reported water levels at plant sites ranging from non-detectable to 550 µg/litre, the highest level being detected in an industrial waste water canal. Vinylidene chloride has also been detected in well and river water from various areas in the USA [200]. Discharge into a sewer is not an acceptable method of disposal for vinylidene chloride. Waste water is therefore injected with steam to allow the vaporization and recovery of vinylidene chloride. Determination of the amount of vinylidene chloride in treated waste water [225] indicated that treatment effected a removal of between 40 and 97%.

In urban storm-water runoff samples in the USA, Cole et al. [30] reported a frequency of detection of vinylidene chloride of 3% when determined among other priority pollutants. The range of detected concentrations was 1.5–4 µg/litre.

Wegman et al., [242] investigated the level of vinylidene chloride present in water from 4 sampling sites in or around a chemical dump that had been used, in particular, for the disposal of by-products

Table 5. Some occupational air exposure limits used in various countries[a]

Country/ Organization	Exposure limit description[b]	Value (mg/m^3)	Effective date[c]
Belgium	Threshold limit value (TLV) - Time-weighted average (TWA) - Short-term exposure limit (STEL)	20 80	1987 (r)
Brazil	Acceptable limit (AC) (48 h/week)	31	1982 (r)
Finland	Time-weighted average (TWA) - Short-term exposure limit (STEL)	40 80	Not given
Germany, Federal Republic of	Maximum work-site concentration (MAK) - Time-weighted average (TWA) - Short-term exposure limit (STEL 30 min)	8 16	1987 (r)
Netherlands	Maximum limit (MXL) - Time-weighted average (TWA) (notice of intended change)	40 20	1987 (r)
Poland	Maximum permissible concentration (MPC) - Ceiling value (CLV)	50	1985 (r)
Romania	Maximum permissible concentration (MPC) - Time-weighted average (TWA) - Ceiling value (CLV)	500 700	1985 (r)

Table 5 (contd).

Sweden	Threshold limit value (TLV)		1985
	- Time-weighted average (TWA)	20	
	- Short-term exposure limit (STEL)	40	
Switzerland	Maximum work-site concentration (MAK)		1987 (r)
	- Time-weighted average (TWA)	8	
United Kingdom	Recommended limit (RECL)		1987 (r)
	- Time-weighted average (TWA)	40	
USA (ACGIH)	Permissible exposure limit (PEL)		1987 (r)
	- Time-weighted average (TWA)	20	
	- Short-term exposure limit (STEL)	80	
USA (NIOSH)	Recommended exposure limit (REL)	lowest reliably detectable concentration	1987 (r)
USSR	Maximum allowable concentration (MAC)		1977
	- Ceiling value (CLV)	50	

[a] From: IRPTC [88].
[b] TWA = A maximum mean exposure limit based generally over the period of a working day (generally 8 or 12 h, except 15 min (Finland) and 30 min (FRG).
 STEL = A maximum concentration of exposure for a specified time duration (generally 15 or 30 min).
[c] When no effective date appears in the IRPTC legal file, the year of the reference from which the data are taken is indicated by (r).

from a pesticide production plant. The levels detected ranged from < 0.01 to 2.8 µg/litre, which compared with levels of 0.3–80 µg/litre reported by the authors to have been detected in the river Rhine.

Concentrations of up to 180 µg/litre were found in ground water beneath a major landfill site in Ottawa, Canada [121]. Low levels of vinylidene chloride have also been observed in other selected contaminated ground waters in Ontario, Canada (Lesage, personal communication, Environment Canada).

Lake Ontario receives the largest burden of industrial and municipal effluents in the Great Lakes Basin with the highly polluted Niagara river contributing 80% of its total inflow. Water samples from 95 stations in Lake Ontario were analysed for a suite of volatile hydrocarbons [104]. Quantifiable amounts of vinylidene chloride were found at 4 stations in the lake (80–190 ng/litre) and a relatively high value of 3500 ng/litre at the fifth station.

In the USSR, the maximum allowable concentration (MAC) of vinylidene chloride in surface water is 0.6 µg/litre [88].

In the study by Lao et al. [115], grab samples of raw sewage and effluents from a sewage treatment plant were found to contain only trace levels of vinylidene chloride (not more than 1 µg/litre). In the same study, ground water from the vicinity of an abandoned waste dump contained a vinylidene chloride (isomer not stated) concentration of 138 µg/litre. The levels of vinylidene chloride in drinking-water were generally non-detectable, the highest detected level being 0.06 µg/litre.

Levels of vinylidene chloride in tap water from Philadelphia and Miami, USA were reported to be 0.1 µg/litre or less [47]. Vinylidene chloride levels were also < 1 µg/litre in raw water supplies at 30 potable water treatment facilities in Canada [163, 164]. In treated water, vinylidene chloride was detected in 1/30 supplies at an average concentration of < 1 µg/litre. The maximum concentration detected in potable water was 20 µg/litre. In the study by Wallace et al., [235] discussed in section 5.1.1, drinking-water samples were also analysed for vinylidene chloride. The median coefficient of variance for analyses was < 10%. Vinylidene chloride was detected occasionally; the percentage of samples that showed measurable concentrations was 26–43 (New

Jersey), 10 (North Carolina), and 0 (North Dakota). The mean concentration in New Jersey drinking-water was measured as 0.1 or 0.2 μg/litre, depending on the year of sampling, and did not exceed 2.5 μg/litre.

Otson [161] reported that vinylidene chloride was detectable in treated (but not untreated) water in only one out of ten municipal water supplies in the lower Great Lakes area of Canada. At this one site, the concentration of vinylidene chloride in treated water was < 0.1 μg/litre. Daily exposure of individuals via the drinking-water in the USA has been estimated at < 0.01 μg, though the maximum could exceed 1 μg [225]. The World Health Organization recommends a maximum concentration of 0.3 μg/litre of drinking-water [88]. The US EPA has proposed a Maximum Contaminant Level (MCL) for vinylidene chloride in drinking-water of 28 μg/litre (7 ppb) [42].

Trace levels of 2 commonly used solvents (trichloroethylene and tetrachloroethylene) have been found in the marine and freshwater environment [104, 130, 231] as well as in ground water. There is an indication that vinylidene chloride may be produced in the degradation of these particular compounds [167, 174], but insufficient data are available to assess the overall importance of trichloroethylene and tetrachloroethylene as sources of vinylidene chloride in the environment.

5.3 Soil

Contamination of the soil may arise through municipal solid waste disposal. It has been estimated that, in the USA, the maximum level of total monomer in the soil does not exceed 81.7 kg (180 pounds) per year [150]. DeLeon et al. [37] investigated the levels of vinylidene chloride in samples from 100 waste-disposal sites. Only one out of three samples from a single site contained a detectable level of vinylidene chloride (21.9 mg/kg dry weight of soil). All remaining samples contained < 10 mg/kg (not detectable).

5.4 Food and Food Packaging

Food may be contaminated by the migration of residual vinylidene chloride monomer from packaging materials containing vinylidene chloride co-polymers.

A number of authors have measured residual levels of vinylidene chloride in commercial food packaging films. A survey of food packaging materials carried out in 1975 in the United Kingdom indicated levels of residual monomer ranging from < 0.001 to 3.8 mg/m^2 [135]. The same group reported residual levels ranging from 0.0003 to 0.4 mg/m^2 from a survey for the period 1977–78. Gilbert et al., [60] reported concentrations of vinylidene chloride monomer ranging from non-detectable (< 0.001 mg/m^2) to 0.022 mg/m^2 in packaging films used for retail foods. Going & Spigarelli [62] reported 4.9 to 58 mg vinylidene chloride/kg (4.9 and 58 ppm) in two samples of Saran wrap while Birkel et al. [18] reported levels of 6.5–26.2 mg/kg (6.5–26.2 ppm). In a study by Hollifield & McNeal [78], vinylidene chloride monomer was detected in commercial food packaging films at 1.6–8.1 mg/kg. However, Tan & Okada [218] and Motegi et al. [144] did not detect vinylidene chloride (< 1 mg/kg) in polyvinylidene chloride film used for fish jelly products, fish sausage, processed cheese, or in household wraps.

Levels of vinylidene chloride reported to migrate into food or food simulants have been quite low. This is consistent with the high barrier properties of vinylidene chloride co-polymers. These co-polymers require little or no added plasticizers to produce flexible films. This has an important effect on their migration characteristics since added plasticizers reduce the barrier properties of polymers. As with any migrant, the amount of vinylidene chloride migration from food packaging depends on the duration of contact, the temperature, and the original concentration in the polymer [142, 170].

Levels of vinylidene chloride were non-detectable (< 5 µg/kg, i.e., < 0.005 ppm) in a range of film packaged foodstuffs except for certain cooked meat products in which the maximum observed concentration was 10 µg/kg (0.001 ppm) [60]. Levels reported for a variety of foods packaged in vinylidene chloride-containing materials ranged from < 1 to 6 μg/kg [135].

Studies on the migration into food simulants carried out by Dow [41] did not show any vinylidene chloride migrating from a vinylidene chloride/vinyl chloride co-polymer film into water (1 h; 212 °F–detection limit 7.5 μg/kg, 7.5 ppb) or into peanut oil (1 h; 212 °F–detection limit 2.5 μg/kg, 2.5 ppb). Migration into heptane (a very efficient extraction solvent) was 13 μg/kg (13 ppb) after 1 h at 180 °F (from a film containing 12 mg residual monomer/kg). A vinylidene chloride/methyl acrylate co-polymer containing residual vinylidene chloride at 9 mg/kg (9 ppm) was extracted with cooking oil at 250 °F for 2 h and then at 120 °F for 15 days. The amount of vinylidene chloride measured in the oil was 18 μg/kg (18 ppb). Extraction with water under the same conditions resulted in 6 μg/litre (6 ppb) migration.

Gas chromatographic determination of sorption isotherms of vinylidene chloride on vinylidene chloride co-polymers by Demertzis et al. [38] was consistent with a strong thermodynamic polymer–monomer interaction leading to a low level of monomer migration from a polymeric package into a food-contacting medium.

It has been estimated that, in the United Kingdom, the maximum possible intake of vinylidene chloride from food as a result of the use of packaging materials is no more than 1 μg/person per day [135].

Proposals for controls on the presence of vinylidene chloride in food-contact materials in the EEC seek to restrict residual vinylidene chloride levels to 5 mg/kg maximum in packaging material and to impose a maximum limit of 50 μg/kg on vinylidene chloride in foods [25]. There is currently no formal regulatory limit on residual vinylidene chloride monomer in food packaging in the USA. The current major USA producer of Saran® has a quality control limit for residual vinylidene chloride in their food packaging film of 10 mg/kg (10 ppm) [41].

Aquatic organisms are a further possible source of contaminated foods. While methods have been developed for analysis of fish tissue [44, 76], no reports of studies on vinylidene chloride levels in fish could be found. However, Ferrario et al. [48] have measured the concentration of vinylidene chloride in biota samples from three passes of Lake Pontchartrain, USA, which serve as a source of aquatic food for human consumption. Vinylidene chloride was not detected in oysters from the Inner Harbour Navigation Canal nor in clams from the Chef Menteur Pass. Clams from the Rigolets Pass contained vinylidene chloride at a concentration of 4.4 µg/kg wet weight.

6. KINETICS AND METABOLISM

6.1 Animals

6.1.1 Absorption

Vinylidene chloride has been shown to be well absorbed via the respiratory and oral routes in mammals. No data are available on dermal absorption.

6.1.1.1 Inhalation exposure

Uptake through inhalation in anaesthetized adult male Sprague-Dawley rats was very rapid, substantial levels being found in venous blood within 2 min of exposure [35]. In this study, calculations of the amount of vinylidene chloride taken up in the body revealed that the cumulative uptake and metabolism of the inhaled chemical was linear for exposures ranging from 100 to 600 mg/m^3 (25 to 150 ppm). There was a trend towards the establishment of equilibrium with saturation of metabolism in the rats exposed to 1200 mg/m^3 (300 ppm), evidenced by levels of vinylidene chloride in the blood and breath, which rose progressively during the last hour of the 3-h exposure. This is in agreement with the approximate saturation of metabolism occurring at the inhalation concentration of 600 mg/m^3 (150 ppm) that Filser & Bolt [49] determined by indirect measurement of vinylidene chloride uptake in male Wistar rats. Andersen et al. [6] found that uptake of vinylidene chloride from a closed chamber occurred in two phases in starved male Holtzmann rats. The rate constant (2.2/h) of the initial rapid phase was independent of initial concentration (40–8000 mg/m^3; 10–2000 ppm) and appeared to represent tissue distribution. Metabolism became nonlinear as dose levels increased (800–4000 mg/m^3; 200–1000 ppm), which is consistent with the findings of Dallas et al. [35] and Filser & Bolt [49] mentioned above.

6.1.1.2 Oral exposure

Jones & Hathaway [102] demonstrated that vinylidene chloride given intragastrically (0.5–350 mg/kg) was completely absorbed from the gastrointestinal tract of Alderley Park (Wistar-derived) male rats. Peak arterial blood levels of orally administered vinylidene chloride (50 mg/kg) were observed within 8 min in male Sprague-Dawley rats [175] and the dose was completely absorbed. Complete absorption of an oral dose of 200 mg/kg to male Sprague-Dawley rats was independent of dose vehicle (aqueous Tween 80, corn oil, or mineral oil) [27]. The vehicle did not affect the half-time for the initial rapid phase of exhalation of vinylidene chloride but the later half-time values were dependent on the rates of absorption, which decreased according to the vehicle in the following order (Tween 80 > corn oil > mineral oil).

6.1.2 Distribution and storage

Whole-body autoradiography revealed that an intragastric dose of [^{14}C]-vinylidene chloride administered to 80-g Alderley Park strain male rats was distributed throughout the tissues of the body within 1 h after initial concentration of the radiolabel in the liver and kidneys, which retained ^{14}C for the longest times after dosing [102]. McKenna et al. [133] also studied the tissue distribution of [^{14}C]-vinylidene chloride following oral dosing (1 or 50 mg/kg) in male Sprague-Dawley rats. Tissue residues, 72 h after dosing, were found in descending order in the liver, kidneys, and other tissues including lung, muscle, skin, blood, and fat.

Similarly, ^{14}C activity derived from inhaled [^{14}C]-vinylidene chloride (exposure concentrations of 40 or 800 mg/m^3 (10 or 200 ppm) for 6 h) in fed male Sprague-Dawley rats (4 animals per group) was also highest in the liver and kidneys, 72 h after termination of exposure. The levels in other tissues at this time showed the following trend: lung > skin > plasma > carcass > muscle and fat [132].

6.1.3 Elimination

The elimination of vinylidene chloride administered intravenously (10–100 mg/kg in 50% polyethylene glycol 400) to fed and fasted male Sprague-Dawley rats followed a tri-exponential pattern corresponding to different half-times and redistribution among tissue compartments. The biological half-life ranged from approximately 40–45 min (10 mg/kg iv) to approximately 55–70 min

(100 mg/kg iv). In orally dosed animals, the half-life values were significantly reduced by fasting suggesting delayed absorption in fed animals [175].

6.1.3.1 Elimination of unchanged vinylidene chloride

As the capacity for the metabolism of vinylidene chloride is subject to saturation (section 6.1.4), the pulmonary elimination of unchanged vinylidene chloride is dose dependent. Male rats given an oral dose of 1 mg/kg, excreted <3% of the dose unchanged via the lung [133]. A similar finding that only 1% of an oral dose (0.5 mg/kg) to rats was eliminated via the pulmonary route was reported by Jones & Hathaway [102]. However, at higher oral dose levels, for example at 350 mg/kg, nearly 70% of the dose was eliminated unchanged via the lungs within 72 h [102]. In a separate study, almost 50% of an oral dose of 200 mg/kg was eliminated via the lungs in rats [27]. The non-linear dose dependency of pulmonary elimination following oral administration, in addition to being influenced by saturable metabolism, is also determined by an efficient transfer of vinylidene chloride from the arteries to the alveoli. Thus, 80% of an intravenous dose of 0.5 mg/kg was eliminated unchanged via the lungs in 1 h. Hence, vinylidene chloride that escapes "first pass" hepatic metabolism is largely removed by pulmonary excretion [102]. Very similar results were obtained by Reichert et al. [184] using female rats. In this study, 1.3, 9.7, or 16.5% of the dose was exhaled within 72 h as unchanged vinylidene chloride after single oral doses of 0.5, 5, or 50 mg/kg, respectively. Fasting of rats for 18 h prior to vinylidene chloride administration (50 mg/kg, oral) led to a reduction in metabolism and consequently a higher level of exhaled unchanged compound [133].

The biphasic pulmonary elimination of [^{14}C]-vinylidene chloride in rats displayed half-lives of 21 and 66 min at an oral dose of 50 mg/kg and approximately 25 and 117 min at an oral dose of 1 mg/kg [133]. When an oral dose of 200 mg/kg was administered to Sprague-Dawley rats, the half-life values for the initial rapid phase ranged from 15 to 21 min and from 10 to 13 min for fasted and fed rats, respectively. The later slow phase of vinylidene chloride exhalation was most prolonged when the compound was administered in mineral oil (respective half-life values of 257 and 280 min), intermediate when it was given in corn oil (73 and 103 min), and shortest (22 and 42 min) when the vehicle was aqueous Tween-80 [27]. Following inhalation of 40 mg [^{14}C]-vinylidene chloride/m^3 (10 ppm), the biphasic pulmonary elimination in rats displayed half-life values of 20 and 217 min for the rapid and slow phases, respectively [132]. As with the oral route, rats exposed to a relatively high dose (800 mg/m^3; 200 ppm) excreted a greater percentage (fed rats 4.7% and fasted rats 8.3%) of their body burden via the lungs than rats exposed to a low exposure of 40 mg/m^3 (10 ppm) (fed rats 1.63% and fasted rats 1.60%). The pharmacokinetics of orally dosed and inhaled vinylidene chloride in fed and fasted rats are illustrated in Fig. 1.

6.1.3.2 Elimination of metabolites

In the studies reported above [102, 133], in which fed rats were dosed orally with 0.5 or 1 mg [^{14}C]-vinylidene chloride/kg, the major route of excretion of metabolites was the urine (63–80% of dose in 3 days). In bile duct-cannulated rats, urinary excretion of ^{14}C was markedly reduced by approximately the same extent as biliary ^{14}C secretion [102]. Hence, approximately half of the urinary metabolites appeared to be derived from the bile following enterohepatic circulation. The lungs were a minor route of elimination of metabolites, 5–14% of the dose was exhaled as carbon dioxide (CO_2). Urine was also the major excretory route for vinylidene chloride metabolites in mice following oral administration [103], only 8–16% of the dose appearing as metabolites in the faeces. This was also the case following intraperitoneal administration. At a higher oral dose level (350 mg/kg), as expected from the saturation of metabolism, a lower level of approximately 30% of the dose appeared as urinary metabolites with less than 1% as CO_2 in expired air and 1.3% in the faeces [102]. Following an intermediate oral dose of 50 mg/kg [133], urinary and faecal elimination were 47% and 4%, respectively, with only 4% exhaled as CO_2. Urinary elimination was biphasic at oral doses of 1 and 50 mg/kg and the initial rapid and terminal phases of urinary elimination displayed half-lives of approximately 6 and 17 h, respectively [133]. Results in female rats were similar to those in males in that 43.6, 53.9, and 42.1% of the dose appeared in the urine

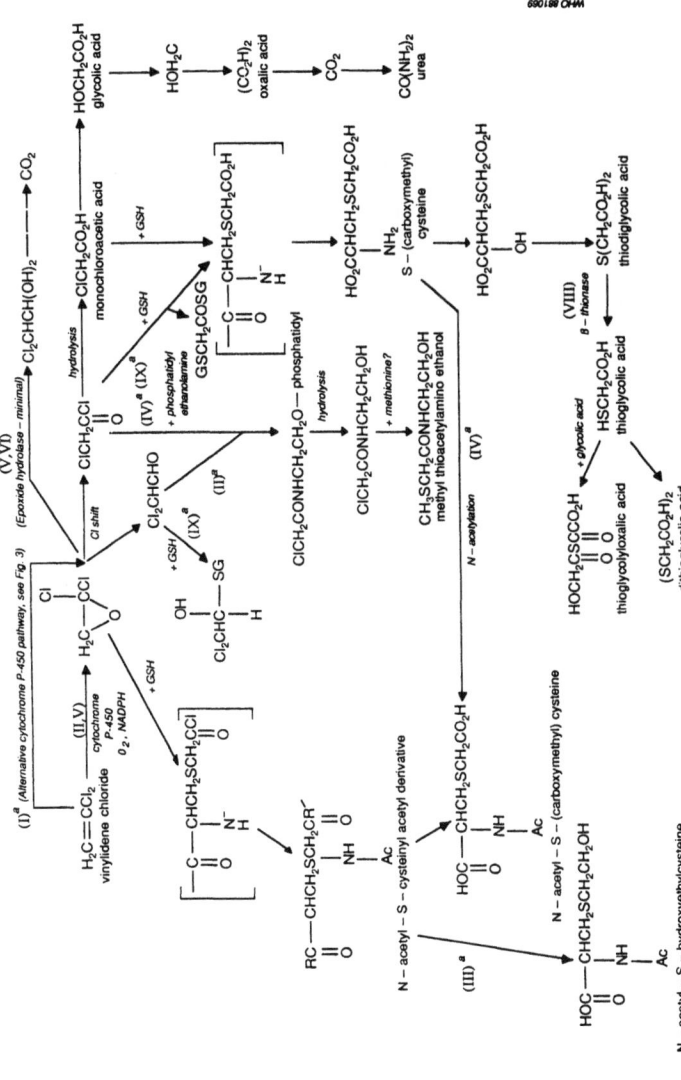

Fig. 2. Scheme for the metabolism of vinylidene chloride in rats, including names of metabolites identified *in vivo*. From Jones & Hathaway [102].
References for additional or alternative pathways that have been suggested giving supportive evidence: (I) Liebler & Guengerich [122], (II) Costa & Ivanetich [32], (III) McKenna et al. [131], (IV) Reichert et al. [184], (V) Leibman & Ortiz [120], (VI) Andersen et al. [7], (VII) Greim et al. [64], (VIII) Jones & Hathaway [103], (IX) Liebler et al. [123, 124].

following oral administration of 0.5, 5, and 50 mg/kg [^{14}C]-vinylidene chloride, respectively. The respective values for CO_2 in expired air were 13.6, 11.4, and 6.1% [184]. Female rats also eliminated metabolites via the faeces (15.7, 14.5, and 7.7% of the dose, respectively), presumably via the biliary route.

Following inhalation of [^{14}C]-vinylidene chloride [132] at 40 mg/m^3 (10 ppm), fed rats excreted 75% of the body burden as urinary metabolites, 8.7% as CO_2 from the lungs, and 9.7% in the faeces. At 800 mg/m^3 (200 ppm), these percentages were slightly lower because a greater proportion of the dose was expired unchanged.

In conclusion, irrespective of the route of administration, the urine is the major route of excretion of metabolites of vinylidene chloride. The extent of elimination by the urine is dependent on dose, since a larger proportion of the dose is eliminated unchanged via the lung at relatively high dose levels, because of the saturation of the metabolism. The efficiency of elimination is such that vinylidene chloride is not expected to accumulate in animals.

6.1.4 Metabolic transformation

The profile of metabolites of vinylidene chloride produced in rats is shown in Fig. 2. This pathway is based on the study by Jones & Hathaway [102] with supportive and, in some cases, conflicting or additional data superimposed. The proportion of vinylidene chloride that is not eliminated unchanged in exhaled air undergoes initial oxidation catalysed by the cytochrome P-450 system. The postulated transient product of this reaction, vinylidene chloride oxide, has escaped isolation because of its instability. This intermediate may be directly conjugated with glutathione or, following an intramolecular rearrangement, conjugated with mono- or bis-glutathione or with phosphatidyl ethanolamine. Monochloroacetic acid may also be formed by hydrolysis and this may be conjugated with glutathione and further metabolized via a pathway involving ß-thionase activity or alternatively may be degraded to CO_2 via glycolic and oxalic acids.

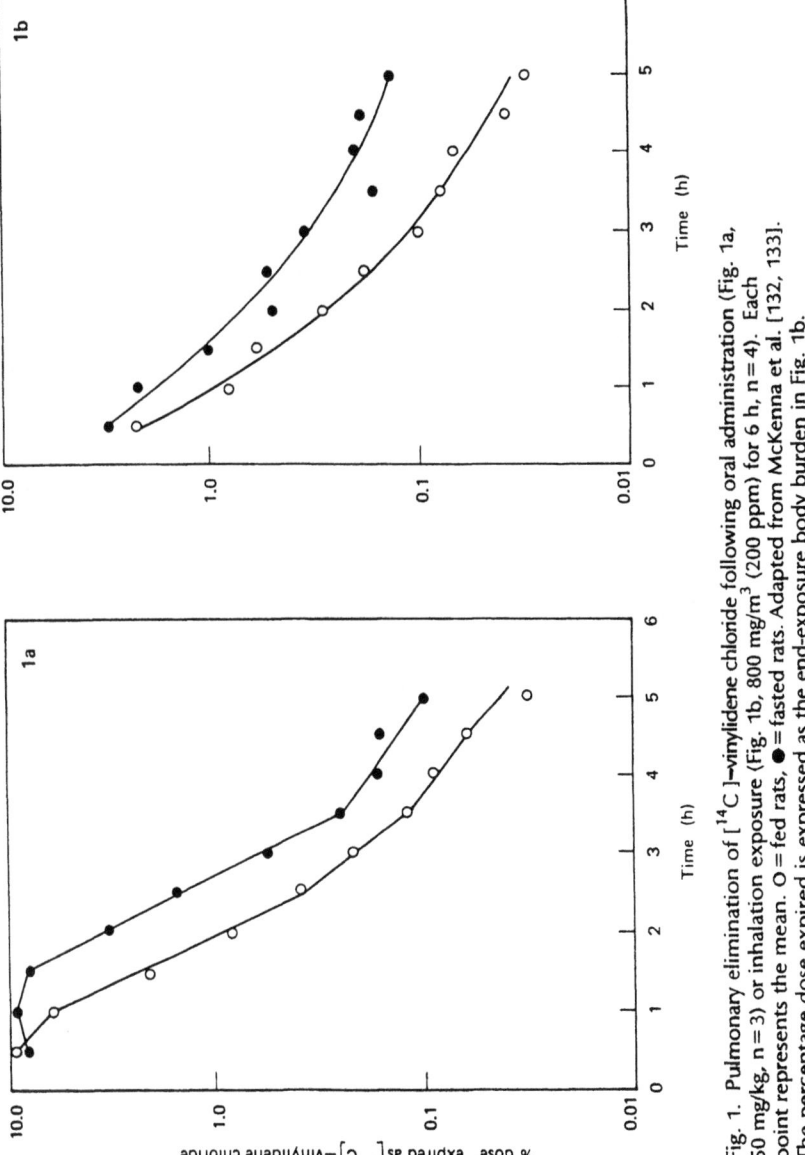

Fig. 1. Pulmonary elimination of [^{14}C]-vinylidene chloride following oral administration (Fig. 1a, 50 mg/kg, n=3) or inhalation exposure (Fig. 1b, 800 mg/m^3 (200 ppm) for 6 h, n=4). Each point represents the mean. O = fed rats, ● = fasted rats. Adapted from McKenna et al. [132, 133]. The percentage dose expired is expressed as the end-exposure body burden in Fig. 1b.

In the study by Jones & Hathaway [102], the metabolic fate of [^{14}C]-vinylidene chloride was investigated in groups of 4 Alderley Park (Wistar derived) male rats. Excreta were analysed for radiolabel following a single intragastric dose of either [1-^{14}C]- or [2-^{14}C]-vinylidene chloride (350 mg/kg). Urinary metabolites were separated by gas chromatography and mass spectra were obtained for major metabolites. The metabolic fate of a single oral dose of [^{14}C]-vinylidene chloride was studied in female Wistar rats by Reichert et al. [184], who also used gas chromatography and mass spectroscopy for the identification of metabolites. The results confirmed the thiodiglycolic acid pathway (Fig. 2) reported by Jones & Hathaway [102]. However, these authors were unable to detect any hydroxyethyl mercapturic acid (Fig. 2), which McKenna et al. [133] had proposed to be a metabolite in male Sprague-Dawley rats on the basis of analysis of the methylated product by mass spectroscopy. A metabolic pathway involving phosphatidyl ethanolamine was uncovered by Reichert et al. [184] by the isolation of the ethanolamine derivative of chloroacetic acid (12% of urinary ^{14}C) (Fig. 2). While this derivative may stem from the reaction of phosphatidyl ethanolamine with chloroacetic acid chloride, it has been proposed by Costa & Ivanetich [32] (see below) that the reaction may be with dichloroacetaldehyde (Fig. 2).

The metabolic fate of vinylidene chloride (50 mg/kg, oral) in Alderley Park male mice is qualitatively very similar to that described for the rat [103]. An exception is the excretion by the mouse (but not the rat) of a small amount of N-acetyl-S- (2-carboxymethyl) cysteine, derived either from the N-acetyl-S-cysteinyl acetyl derivative or from S-(carboxymethyl) cysteine, which are common to both species. Quantitative differences between the metabolites formed in the two species are shown in Table 6. It is seen that mice metabolized 22% more of the administered dose than rats and, consequently, released less unchanged vinylidene chloride in the expired air. The species difference was attributed to higher cytochrome P-450-mediated epoxidation in mice. The quantitative difference in the proportion of the N-acetyl-S-cysteinyl acetyl derivative correlates with that expected on the basis of hepatic glutathione-S-epoxide transferase activity in these species, and may also be influenced by the lower extent of chloro- acetic acid metabolism in mice. Exposure to 40 mg [^{14}C]-vinylidene

Table 6. Relative proportion of ^{14}C excretory products after oral administration of [1-^{14}C]-vinylidene chloride to rodents at 50 mg/kg [a]

[^{14}C] Excretory products	% of ^{14}C dose	
	Mice	Rats
Pulmonary excretion		
Unchanged vinylidene chloride	6	28
CO_2	3	3.5
Urinary excretion		
Chloroacetic acid	0	1
Thiodiglycollic acid	3	22
Thioglycollic acid	5	3
Dithioglycollic acid	23	5
Thioglycollyloxalic acid	3	2
N-Acetyl-S-cysteinyl acetyl derivative	50	28
N-Acetyl-S-(2-carboxymethyl) cysteine	4	
Urea	3	3.5

[a] From: Jones & Hathway [103].

chloride/m^3 (10 ppm) for 6 h resulted in a body burden of 5.3 mg equivalents/kg in male Ha (ICR) mice compared with 2.9 mg equivalents/kg in male Sprague-Dawley rats [131]. Since only 0.65 and 1.63% of the dose were recovered respectively, as unchanged vinylidene chloride, it was concluded that total metabolism was more efficient in the mouse, as reported by Jones & Hathway [103].

Recent studies by Liebler & Guengerich [122] confirmed the hydrolytic lability of vinylidene chloride oxide, which was chemically synthesized and characterized by nuclear magnetic resonance and mass spectroscopy. Selectivity was observed between purified rat liver cytochrome P-450s in the production of Cl_2CHCHO and P-450 inactivation but not in glycolic acid ($ClCH_2CO_2H$) production. Further, aqueous decomposition of vinylidene chloride did not produce Cl_2CHCHO and yielded glycolic acid only at low pH. These data, coupled with kinetic studies of vinylidene chloride oxidation, suggest that vinylidene chloride oxide is not an obligate intermediate in Cl₂CHCHO and ClCH₂CO₂H production. A proposed scheme for the role of cytochrome P-450 is shown in Fig. 3. Whether or not this scheme operates *in vivo*, is uncertain.

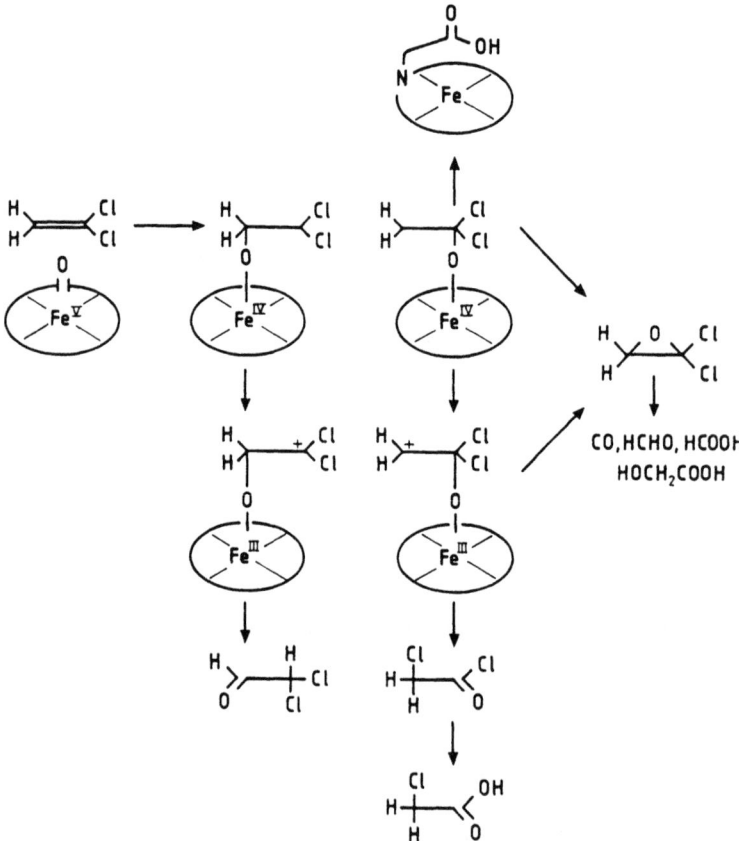

Fig. 3. A possible route for the *in vitro* oxidation of vinylidene chloride by cytochrome P-450. Modified from Liebler & Guengerich [122].

N.B. It is not known whether this pathway occurs *in vivo*.

The role of cytochrome P-450 in the metabolism of vinylidene chloride was confirmed by the measurement of a Type I difference spectrum with the bound substrate in hepatic microsomes from male Long-Evans rats [32]. Addition of vinylidene chloride to microsomes also stimulated carbon monoxide-inhibitable NADPH oxidation. NADPH was required for the conversion of vinylidene chloride to monochloroacetic acid and dichloroacetaldehyde (not found in the *in vivo* studies reported above), and these metabolites were not formed in the presence of cytochrome P-450 inhibitors SKF-525A and carbon monoxide. Pretreatment of rats with the cytochrome P-450-inducing agent ß-naphthoflavone did not elevate the hepatic microsomal metabolism of vinylidene chloride, and the cytochrome P-450-inducing agent phenobarbital gave a slight enhancement of metabolism per mg microsomal protein. More noticeable was the marked enhancement of the ability of liver preparations to produce mutagenic metabolites of vinylidene chloride *in vitro* following treatment of female BD-VI rats with the selective inducing agents phenobarbital and 3-methylcholanthrene [15].

In a study by Sato et al. [195], male Wistar rats were given ethanol in the diet (2% ethanol, increased by 1% daily to a final concentration of 5%, equivalent to 30% of total calorie intake). Hepatic microsomes derived from the ethanol-treated rats metabolized vinylidene chloride at a rate of 100.6 nmol/g liver per min compared with 31.1 nmol/g liver per min in control rat microsomes, indicating induction of microsomal enzymes involved in vinylidene chloride metabolism.

As shown in Fig. 2, conjugation with glutathione required prior microsomal metabolism of vinylidene chloride [131]. The importance of glutathione in vinylidene chloride metabolism was studied by Andersen et al. [7]. Pretreatment of rats with agents that deplete hepatic non-protein sulfhydryl concentrations caused a marked inhibition of vinylidene chloride metabolism as measured by gas uptake (which is determined by metabolism). In particular, treatment with cyclohexene oxide and dimethylmaleate resulted in 76 and 54% inhibition, respectively. Reichert et al. [183] also noted an 18% reduction in the metabolism of vinylidene chloride (given as 20 000 mg/m^3 (5000 ppm) in the gaseous phase) in isolated perfused rat livers following diethylmaleate administration. This was considered to be due to an 85% reduction in glutathione levels. The finding that the glutathione conjugate ClCH$_2$COSG is able to

S-alkylate a second glutathione molecule to yield GSCH$_2$COSG [123, 124] suggests that the monoglutathione conjugate may have the ability to interact with proteins, such as those involved in the transport of glutathione conjugates.

The rate of metabolism of vinylidene chloride by isolated hepatocytes from phenobarbital-pretreated male Long-Evans rats was studied by Costa & Ivanetich [33] using the maximum dose of vinylidene chloride that was not cytotoxic (2.1 mmol vinylidene chloride/litre). The metabolites detected were dichloroacetic acid (0.15 nmol/10^6 cells per 10 min), monochloroacetic acid (0.068 nmol/10^6 cells per 60 min), and dichloroethanol (0.01 nmol/10^6 cells per 10 min). 2-Chloroethanol and chloroacetaldehyde were not detected (<12 and <4 nmol/10^6 cells per 30 min, respectively). No attempt was made to hydrolyse conjugates.

In summary, the phase I metabolism of vinylidene chloride in rodents involves the action of cytochrome P-450 and the production of monochloroacetic acid. This, and its precursors, may undergo conjugation with glutathione and/or phosphatidyl ethanolamine prior to further conversions. Metabolism in the mouse occurs at a greater rate than in the rat and results in a similar metabolic profile with a relatively higher proportion of glutathione conjugate derivatives.

6.1.5 Reaction with cellular macromolecules

The specific interaction of vinylidene chloride metabolite(s) with DNA is covered in section 8.5.1.

In the studies by McKenna et al. [132, 133] reported in section 6.1.3.1, fasted rats showed a reduced capacity to metabolize relatively high doses of both orally administered and inhaled [^{14}C]-vinylidene chloride. Fasted rats exposed to 800 mg vinylidene chloride/m^3 (200 ppm) sustained liver and kidney damage, which was not found in fed rats. This toxicity was associated with a greater level of covalently bound radiolabel in the liver of the fasted animals. An elevated level of covalent binding in the liver was also seen as a result of depriving rats of food prior to administration of an oral dose of 50 mg vinylidene chloride/kg. The results can be explained by the binding of reactive metabolites (presumed to be vinylidene chloride oxide and/or chloroacetyl chloride) to nucleophilic sites in tissue macromolecules. This is thought to be enhanced by the depletion of glutathione during fasting [93], which operates as an alternative nucleophile [131]. Following exposure of male rats to 20–800 mg [^{14}C]-vinylidene chloride/m^3 (5–200 ppm) for 6 h [131], hepatic non-protein sulfhydryl levels fell in a dose-dependent saturable manner. Appreciable covalent binding of radiolabel to hepatic protein occurred when 30% or more glutathione was depleted. Covalent binding of radiolabel to hepatic and kidney tissue in mice occurred at the rate of 22 and 80 μg equivalents/g protein, respectively, compared with 5 and 13 μg equivalents/g protein, respectively, in rat tissue following exposure to 40 mg [^{14}C]-vinylidene chloride /m^3 (10 ppm) for 6 h.

In a separate study on rats by Reichert et al. [183], the rate of depletion of glutathione after oral doses of vinylidene chloride was also found to be exponentially dependent on the concentration. However, the authors questioned the correlation between a low glutathione level and relatively high toxicity in fasted rats, since the fall in glutathione levels after oral administration of vinylidene chloride (1000 mg/kg) was identical in fasted rats and fed rats. Furthermore, the rate of metabolism of vinylidene chloride by isolated perfused livers (20 000 mg vinylidene chloride/m^3 (5000 ppm) in the gaseous phase) was not affected by an 18-h fast. The interpretation of these data is difficult in the light of other results reported in this section.

Jaeger et al. [93] reported a diurnal variation in the levels of glutathione in male Holtzmann rats. The animals were most sensitive to the lethal and hepatotoxic effects of vinylidene chloride when glutathione levels were at a minimum. Jaeger et al. [96] also correlated susceptibility to the hepatotoxicity of vinylidene chloride (exposure for 4 h at 4000 mg/m^3 (1000 ppm)) to decreased hepatic glutathione concentrations in male Holtzmann rats that had been fasted for 18 h or had been treated with diethylmaleate. In a further study [97], the hepatic glutathione concentration was decreased by the administration of trichloropropane epoxide (0.1 ml of a 10% solution/kg) to fasted rats. This treatment was also associated with elevated toxicity of vinylidene chloride. A qualitative, but not a quantitative, difference in the metabolism of vinylidene chloride

(8000 mg/m^3 (2000 ppm) initial exposure) resulted from the fasting of rats. Thirty minutes after exposure to [^{14}C]-vinylidene chloride at the same concentration, the radioactivity in liver mitochondria and microsomes was largely TCA-insoluble and was greater in fasted than in control rats. Judging from the turn-over time of TCA-insoluble ^{14}C, it was suggested that this ^{14}C had entered the metabolic pool rather than being covalently bound to macromolecules. However, the demonstration of labile thiol adducts [123] could explain this finding.

Covalent binding of [1,2-^{14}C]-vinylidene chloride to tissues peaked 6 h after an intraperitoneal dose of 125 mg/kg in male C57B1/6N mice [159]. Pretreatment with diethylmaleate, which depletes glutathione, enhanced covalent binding in the liver, lung, and kidney, and also enhanced lethal toxicity. In accordance with evidence for the formation of reactive metabolites of vinylidene chloride by cytochrome P-450, covalent binding was increased in liver and lung tissue by pretreatment with the P-450 inducers, phenobarbital and 3-methylcholanthrene. Inhibitors of cytochrome P-450, piperonyl butoxide, and SKF-525A all decreased covalent binding in the liver and lung. However, binding to kidney tissue was not affected by P-450-inducing agents, was decreased by piperonyl butoxide and was increased by SKF-525A. Covalent binding occurred in hepatic and lung microsomes from these mice following incubation of microsomes with NADPH. Surprisingly, however, oxygen did not appear to be necessary. Kidney microsomes could not metabolize vinylidene chloride to products that covalently bound to tissue macromolecules, unless the mice had been pretreated with cytochrome P-450-inducing agents suggesting that, in the absence of enzyme induction, covalent binding in the kidney *in vivo* was mediated by hepatic metabolites [157, 158]. Covalent binding of [^{14}C]-vinylidene chloride to lung and liver tissue accompanied bronchiolar necrosis in CD-1 mice given an intraperitoneal dose (125 mg/kg); only mild hepatic necrosis was observed ([56]–section 8.1.3.1). The effects of various inducers and inhibitors of cytochrome P-450 activity on toxicity and covalent binding were variable in line with the evidence for microsomal-mediated activation and deactivation (section 8.1.2) and in accordance with multiple reactive metabolites (see below). Vinylidene chloride epoxide, 2-chloroacetyl chloride, 2,2-dichloroacetaldehyde, 2-chloroacetic acid and S-(2-chloroacetyl)-glutathione all bind covalently to thiols *in vitro* [123, 124]. Covalent binding of radiolabel to microsomal protein occurred following incubation of [^{14}C]-vinylidene chloride with rat and human liver microsomes. When rat microsomes were used, binding was inhibited by alcohol dehydrogenase + NADH, suggesting that 2,2-dichloroacetaldehyde played a role in the binding process. Metabolites of [^{14}C]-vinylidene chloride bound to microsomes from isolated lung as well as from the liver of CD-1 mice [54]. By the use of specific inhibitors and agents that induce cytochrome P-450 isoenzymes, these authors were able to demonstrate the role of cytochrome P-450 isoenzymes in the production of reactive metabolites, though some non-specific covalent binding was also seen.

In summary, there are a number of reactive metabolites of vinylidene chloride, the production of which is dependent on the activity of cytochrome P-450. In rodents, each of these products may contribute to the depletion of glutathione and to covalent binding to tissue macromolecules, which is greater in the liver than in the kidney. The greater covalent binding of reactive metabolites to tissue macromolecules in the mouse compared with the rat is correlated with a relatively higher rate of metabolism (section 6.1.4) and higher toxicity (section 8.1.1.2).

6.1.6 Transformation by non-mammalian species

No data were available to the Task Group on vinylidene chloride metabolism in non-mammalian species, other than bacteria.

6.2 Human Beings

No data have been reported on the kinetics and metabolism of vinylidene chloride in human beings, other than some very limited information obtained indirectly through the following studies. Liver 9000-g supernatants (S9) from four adults, who did not show any pathological lesions, were capable of catalysing the formation of products that were mutagenic to *Salmonella typhimurium* [15] (section 8.5.2), suggesting that human cytochrome P-450 can metabolize vinylidene chloride. The rate of conversion of vinylidene chloride to dichloroacetaldehyde in hepatic microsomes from two human organ donors (one of each sex) was 0.034–0.038 nmol/min per nmol cytochrome P-450. The conversion was shown (by lack of significant antibody inhibition) not to be mediated by debrisoquine hydroxylase (a form of cytochrome P-450, which is polymorphic in human beings) [245]. This rate of microsomal metabolism to dichloroacetaldehyde is similar to that reported by Costa & Ivanetich [33] for the rat (0.028 nmol dichloroacetaldehyde and 0.035 nmol chloroacetate produced/min per nmol cytochrome P-450).

Vinylidene chloride is exhaled in human breath following inhalation exposure [233]. Breath from student volunteers, in Texas and North Carolina, USA, was sampled using a spirometer as the subjects inhaled pure air. The ratio of vinylidene chloride in the breath to that in pre-exposure air was 0.78 ± 0.86 (n = 15). A significant Spearman correlation coefficient of 0.77 was determined between air and breath levels of vinylidene chloride in 17 human subjects. The following log-linear model was capable of giving a reasonable prediction of breath levels from the preceding 8-h air exposure levels: log concentration in breath ($\mu g/m^3$) = -0.24 ± 0.67 + (0.71 ± 0.17) log concentration in air ($\mu g/m^3$). The authors suggested that, if these observations were confirmed, recent exposures and body burdens of individuals could be estimated from breath analysis. However, this may be hampered by biphasic elimination as reported for animals (section 6.1.3).

7. EFFECTS ON ORGANISMS IN THE ENVIRONMENT

7.1 Effects on the Stratospheric Ozone Layer

The rapid destruction of vinylidene chloride in the troposphere by hydroxyl radicals (section 4.1.1) indicates that the substance is unlikely to participate in the depletion of the stratospheric ozone layer.

7.2 Aquatic Organisms

Studies on the impact of vinylidene chloride on living organisms have concentrated on the aquatic environment and include discussions on the levels of vinylidene chloride detected (section 5.2).

According to Leblanc [117], the acute toxicity for the water flea (*Daphnia magna*), under static conditions, is of a similar magnitude to that reported by Buccafusco et al. [21] for the bluegill fish (see below). The median LC_{50} values were 98 mg/litre (95% confidence interval; range, 71–130 mg/litre) and 79 mg/litre (95% confidence interval; range, 61–110 mg/litre) for 24 h and 48 h, respectively. The "no discernible effect" level for the water flea was less than 2.4 mg/litre.

Dawson et al. [36] treated fresh-water bluegill sunfish (*Lepomis macrochiras*) and marine tidewater silverside fish (*Menidia beryllina*) with vinylidene chloride (132–750 mg/litre and 180–320 mg/litre, respectively) for up to 96 h under static conditions. No attempt was made to prevent loss of vinylidene chloride by evaporation. The best-fit median lethal concentrations (LC_{50}) for 96 h were 220 and 250 mg/litre for bluegill sunfish and tidewater silverside fish, respectively. Since these values were less than 500 mg/litre (500 ppm), vinylidene chloride was designated a hazardous substance. The 96-h static LC_{50} of vinylidene chloride in juvenile marine sheepshead minnows (*Cyprinodon variegatus*) was very similar to the above values (250 mg/litre; range, 200–340 mg/litre, 95% confidence limits), and was the same when measured at 24 h [72]. The no-observed-effect concentration was

80 mg/litre. The acute toxicity in bluegill fish (*L. macrochirus*) was also investigated by Buccafusco et al. [2] under static conditions, in capped jars to minimize volatilization. The recorded LC_{50} value was 74 mg/litre (95% confidence interval, 57–91 mg/litre) at 96 h. This LC_{50}, which was identical at 24 h, is somewhat lower than those reported in the studies by Dawson et al. [36] and Heitmuller et al. [72]. Toxicity values similar to those noted above for fish and *Daphnia* were reported in a review by Atri [9].

The assays under static uncapped conditions reported here are relevant to acute spill conditions. One-week flow-through studies have also been carried out by Dill et al. [39]. The LC_{50} value for fathead minnows (*Pimephales promelas* Rafinesque) in flowing water was 29 mg/litre (range, 23–34 mg/litre) after 7 days exposure, whereas the 96-h LC_{50} was 108 mg/litre (range, 85–117 mg/litre) under flow-through conditions. Swimming disorientation was observed to be the major sublethal toxic effect of vinylidene chloride. A bioconcentration factor of 4 and a bioaccumulation factor of 6.9 have been reported for fish in a review by Atri [9].

Few data are available on the sublethal effects of vinylidene chloride on aquatic organisms. Preliminary studies demonstrated that hepatic neoplastic lesions were not produced in guppy (*Poecilia reticulata*) and Japanese medaka (*Oryzias latipes*) exposed to vinylidene chloride concentrations of up to 40 mg/litre (40 ppm) for 3 months [71] (personal communication, Hawkins Gulf Coast Research Laboratory, Mississippi, USA).

8. EFFECTS ON EXPERIMENTAL ANIMALS AND *IN VITRO* TEST SYSTEMS

8.1 Single Exposures

Acute toxicity data (LC_{50}s and LD_{50}s) for common laboratory animals are shown in Table 7.

8.1.1 Inhalation

8.1.1.1 Rats

In an early study by Carpenter et al. [24], 3 groups of 6 Sherman rats were exposed to vinylidene chloride vapour for 4 h at various concentrations. Within a 14-day post-exposure observation period, a concentration of 128 000 mg/m^3 (32 000 ppm) was lethal for 2/6, 3/6, and 4/6 animals, respectively. Later, Siegel et al. [206] estimated a 4-h LC_{50} of 25 400 mg vinylidene chloride/m^3 (6350 ppm) for groups of 16 male Sprague-Dawley-derived rats.

Siletchnik & Carlson [211] considered that lethality from vinylidene chloride might be related to cardiotoxicity. They exposed male Charles River albino rats to 102 400 mg vinylidene chloride/m^3 (25 600 ppm) for 10 min or more and noted progressive sinus bradycardia and arrhythmias (AV-block), multiple continuous ventricular contractions, and ventricular fibrillation. This treatment with vinylidene chloride also produced a marked increase in sensitivity to epinephrine-induced cardiac arrhythmias. Phenobarbital pretreatment enhanced the cardiac-sensitizing properties of vinylidene chloride.

However, Jaeger et al. [95] reported that death from vinylidene chloride inhalation was associated with bloody ascites in all animals, with no signs of cardiac failure, and was therefore thought to be due to vascular collapse and shock.

In the studies by Zeller et al. [248, 249], the estimated LC_{50}s of vinylidene chloride (Table 7) were lowered by fasting in both male and female Sprague-Dawley rats. Females were less susceptible

Table 7. Acute toxicity of vinylidene chloride for laboratory animals

Species	Sex	Nutritional status	Estimated LC_{50}/LD_{50}	Dosing criteria	Limit of observation time	Reference
Rat	male, female	fed	approximately 128 000 mg/m^3 (32 000 ppm)	Inhalation, 4 h	14 days	[24]
Rat	male	fed	25 400 mg/m^3 (6350 ppm)	Inhalation, 4 h	14 days	[206]
Rat	male	fed	60 000 mg/m^3 (15 000 ppm)	Inhalation, 4 h	24 h	[96]
Rat	male	fed	approximately 8000 mg/m^3 (2000 ppm)	inhalation, 4 h (pm but not am)	23 h	[93]
Rat	male	fed	28 400 mg/m^3 (7100 ppm)	Inhalation, 4 h	14 days	[249]
Rat	male	18-h fasted	2400 mg/m^3 (600 ppm)	Inhalation, 4 h	24 h	[96]
Rat	male	fasted (overnight)	not measurable because of non-linear concentration–mortality relationship	inhalation, 4 h		[5]
Rat	male	16-h fasted	1660 mg/m^3 (415 ppm)	Inhalation, 4 h	14 days	[248]
Rat	female	fed	41 200 mg/m^3 (10 300 ppm)	Inhalation, 4 h	14 days	[249]
Rat	female	16-h fasted	26 260 mg/m^3 (6565 ppm)	Inhalation, 4 h	14 days	[248]

Table 7 (contd).

Mouse	male female	fed	392 mg/m³ (98 ppm) 420 mg/m³ (105 ppm)	inhalation, 1 day	[204]
Mouse	male	fed	140 mg/m³ (35 ppm)	Inhalation, 2 days	[204]
Mouse	male	fed	460 mg/m³ (115 ppm)	Inhalation, 4 h	14 days	[251]
Mouse	male	fasted	200 mg/m³ (50 ppm)	Inhalation, 4 h	14 days	[250]
Mouse	female	fed	820 mg/m³ (205 ppm)	Inhalation, 4 h	14 days	[251]
Mouse	female	fasted	500 mg/m³ (125 ppm)	Inhalation, 4 h	14 days	[250]
Hamster	male	fed	6640 mg/m³ (1660 ppm)	Inhalation, 4 h	14 days	[109]
Hamster	male	fasted	600 mg/m³ (150 ppm)	Inhalation, 4 h	14 days	[108]
Hamster	female	fed	11 780 mg/m³ (2945 ppm)	Inhalation, 4 h	14 days	[109]
Hamster	female	fasted	1780 mg/m³ (445 ppm)	Inhalation, 4 h	14 days	[108]
Rat	male	fed	1550 mg/kg	gavage	24 h	[100]
Rat	male	fed	1510 mg/kg	gavage	96 h	[100]

Table 7 (contd).

Species	Sex	Nutritional status	Estimated LC_{50}/LD_{50}	Dosing criteria	Limit of observation time	Reference
Rat	male	fed	1800 mg/kg	gavage	not stated	[172]
Rat	female	fed	1500 mg/kg	gavage	not stated	[172]
Rat	male	fed	800–2000 mg/kg	gavage	14 days	[2]
Mouse	male	fed	201–235 mg/kg	gavage	not stated	[103]
Mouse	female	fed	171–221 mg/kg	gavage	not stated	[103]

[a] This report noted that mortality was consistently observed at doses as low as 50 mg/kg. In 73-g male rats, dose-mortality curves showed a maximum mortality (10/10) at 300 mg/kg. Percent mortality then decreased as dose was increased to 800 mg/kg.

than males to the lethal effect. Post-mortem examination of animals dying from vinylidene chloride exposure revealed acute contraction of heart blood vessels, acute swellings and localized bloody oedema in the lung, greyish enlarged liver lobules, and pale kidneys. Ascites and hydrothorax were also seen.

Jaeger et al. [96] showed that the toxicity of vinylidene chloride in male Holtzman rats was enhanced as a result of fasting. The estimated 24-h LC_{50} for fed rats was 60 000 mg/m^3 (15 000 ppm) (4-h exposure), while the corresponding value for 18-h fasted rats was 2400 mg/m^3 (600 ppm) (n = 5 or 6). The minimum lethal concentrations were 40 000 and 800 mg/m^3 (10 000 and 200 ppm), respectively. At levels of 600 mg/m^3 (150 ppm) or more, serum-alanine-α-ketoglutarate transaminase rose rapidly in fasted rats (within 2 h of termination of a 4-h exposure at 8000 mg/m^3 (2000 ppm)). This indication of liver damage did not arise at levels below 8000 mg/m^3 (2000 ppm) in rats provided with food. The increased susceptibility of fasted rats was considered to be due to decreased availability of hepatic glutathione and this was supported by the potentiation of hepatotoxicity by treatment of fed rats with the agent diethylmaleate, which depletes glutathione (section 6.1.5). This was further supported by the observation [93] that a 4-h exposure of male Holtzman rats to 8000 mg vinylidene chloride/m^3 (2000 ppm) in the morning produced a 3-fold increase in serum alanine-α-ketoglutarate transaminase activity with no deaths. Conversely, the same treatment in the afternoon resulted in an almost 10-fold increase in serum alanine-α-ketoglutarate transaminase, and 2 out of 5 treated rats died within 23 h. The relative susceptibilities were inversely related to hepatic glutathione levels.

In fasted male Sprague-Dawley rats exposed to 800 mg vinylidene chloride/m^3 (0.02%), liver toxicity was observed within 2 h [188]. Toxicity in liver parenchyma was characterized by retraction of cell borders and the formation of pericellular "lacunae". Nuclei showed segregation of chromatin towards the margins of the nuclear envelope and mitochondria were swollen with ruptured outer membranes. Midzonal hepatic necrosis led to haemorrhagic centrilobular necrosis within 6 h. This liver necrosis, along with raised levels of serum-alanine-α-ketoglutarate transaminase and an associated fall in hepatic glutathione levels, were all minimized by pretreatment of rats with the cytochrome P-450-inducing agents phenobarbital and Aroclor-1254.

In an earlier study [23], male Sprague-Dawley rats were exposed to 5760 mg vinylidene chloride/m^3 (1440 ppm) for 1 h. Twenty-four hours later, liver damage was detected by measured elevations in serum glutamic oxalacetic transaminase and glutamic pyruvic transaminase. Pretreatment of these animals with phenobarbital and 3-methylcholanthrene did not alter the extent of the elevation of serum hepatic enzyme levels. Furthermore, the activity of glucose-6-phosphatase in the liver was also unaffected 24 h after exposure to 9080 or 11 960 mg vinylidene chloride/m^3 (2270 ppm or 2990 ppm) in both 3-methylcholanthrene and phenobarbital-treated animals. In contrast, exposure to 80 000 or 130 000 mg vinylidene chloride/m^3 (20 000 or 32 500 ppm) for 1 h was lethal for most of the rats (groups of 4 rats) pretreated with the inducing agents, despite the fact that these concentrations did not produce deaths in similar groups of control rats. Treatment of rats with the cytochrome P-450 inhibitors "SKF-525A" and "Lilly 18947" reduced the survival time after inhalation of 168 000 or 212 000 mg vinylidene chloride/m^3 (42 000 ppm or 53 000 ppm). Because of the differential effects of inducing agents on hepatotoxicity and lethality, the results suggest that the lethal effects of inhaled vinylidene chloride are distinct from the hepatotoxic effects. Since cytochrome P-450 has been implicated in the activation of vinylidene chloride to form toxic metabolite(s) (section 6.1.4) the protective or lack of potentiating effect of inducing agents on hepatotoxicity is not understood, but may result from multiple roles of microsomal enzymes (section 8.1.2.1).

Subsequently, Reynolds et al. [189] exposed fasted male rats to 800 mg vinylidene chloride/m^3 (200 ppm). Glutathione levels in the liver were rapidly depleted during the first and second hours of exposure and were replenished during the third and fourth hours, when toxicity was determined by analysis of tissue sections by light microscopy. The rebound of glutathione levels was not observed in the mitochondria, which might indicate a role of this organelle in toxicity. Inactivation of the microsomal enzyme cytochrome P-450 was not appreciable prior to histological alterations in the liver and therefore did not appear to be an early event in cytotoxicity. The toxicity of vinylidene chloride (2000 or 4000 mg/m^3 (500 or 1000 ppm)) inhaled for 3 or 24 h was exacerbated by the glutathione-depleting agent phorone, as evidenced by an increase in the levels of serum-aminotransferases and sorbitol dehydrogenase at 3 h and mortality at 24 h in male Wistar rats [207]. Phorone (250 mg/kg) also had the effect of increasing the half-life of the terminal elimination phase of vinylidene chloride from 0.89 to 2.33 h and from 1.55 to 4.21 h at levels of 2000 and 4000 mg vinylidene chloride/m^3 (500 and 1000 ppm), respectively, in a closed exposure chamber. Therefore, increased toxicity was associated with decreased metabolism. Since there was no evidence for an effect of phorone on the activity of the mixed-function oxidase, the authors proposed that phorone produced a quantitative change in vinylidene chloride metabolism leading to intermediates of greater toxicity. However, the results might also be explained by a build up of intermediates (due to reduced ability to conjugate with glutathione) that inhibit their own formation.

Andersen et al. [5] studied the dependence of inhalation toxicity (as measured by plasma aspartate transaminase) on both exposure concentration and duration in fasted male HOT:SD(BR) Holtzman rats. Plasma-enzyme levels increased markedly after exposure to 800 mg vinylidene chloride/m^3 (200 ppm) for 1.25 h. After this time, no further increase in plasma aspartate transaminase was recorded. The concentration–mortality curve increased rapidly between 400 and 800 mg/m^3 (100–200 ppm) and reached a plateau between 800 and 4000 mg/m^3 (200–1000 ppm), making it impossible to make a meaningful estimate of the LC$_{50}$. Thus, a concentration × time relationship for toxicity is not apparent, and this is in agreement with saturable metabolism (section 6.1.3.1) to toxic intermediates. Thus, estimates by other workers of the LC$_{50}$ under similar conditions cannot be considered accurate.

After inhalation of 800 mg vinylidene chloride/m^3 (200 ppm) for 0.5 h, immature rats showed significant prolongation of pentobarbital-induced sleeping times, suggesting an inhibition of pentobarbital metabolism [5]. This increase in sleeping times was maintained for at least 3 days after a 2-h exposure. In mature rats, treated with 1600 mg/m^3 (400 ppm) for 2 h, there was no evidence of an altered sleeping time within the exposure period, though this was elevated 2 and 24 h later.

Exposure of fasted male rats to 8000 mg vinylidene chloride/m^3 (2000 ppm) for 4 h led not only to elevation of serum alanine α-ketoglutarate transaminase levels but also to increased levels of hepatic sodium and calcium with a concomitant decrease in potassium and magnesium levels and diminished histochemical glucose-6-phosphatase activity. These changes were associated with centrilobular necrosis and haemorrhagic necrosis of the entire hepatic lobule. Thyroidectomized, fasted rats, exposed under the same conditions, showed significantly less change in hepatic electrolyte concentrations. Morphological injury was also minimized and was similar to that seen in non-pretreated fed animals. Mortality was also inhibited by thyroidectomy. In contrast, thyroxine pretreatment potentiated the toxicity of vinylidene chloride and restored the susceptibility of thyroidectomized rats. It was suggested that the protective effect of thyroidectomy was at least partially mediated by the observed elevation of hepatic glutathione levels [216].

However, differences were observed between fed, fasted, and hyperthyroid Sprague-Dawley rats in the effects of orally administered vinylidene chloride (50 mg/kg body weight) on body temperature, serum glucose concentrations, hepatic glutathione, and glutathione transferase [106]. The different patterns of response in the three groups suggest different mechanisms of toxicity in fasted and hyperthyroid rats.

Similar findings were reported by Jaeger et al. [98]. In a study on male Sprague-Dawley rats, a raised serum sorbitol dehydrogenase level (a cytoplasmic marker) coincided with an elevation in serum ornithine carbamoyl transaminase from the mitochondria. This finding suggests that mitochondrial damage is an early event in the hepatotoxicity of vinylidene chloride. The data support the authors' theory that the metabolite monochloracetic acid is toxic to mitochondria via chlorocitric acid and "lethal synthesis" leading to accumulation of citric acid [97].

The kidney is also affected by vinylidene chloride. At sublethal concentrations (800 mg/m^3 (200 ppm) for 6 h), male Sprague-Dawley rats given food *ad libitum* did not show any signs of an adverse response [132]. In contrast, rats previously fasted for 18 h, were found to have haemoglobinuria, which persisted for

12–24 h after exposure. As well as seeing multiple foci of hepatic centrilobular degeneration and necrosis, marked degeneration of kidney proximal tubular epithelia was observed after this exposure in the fasted rats, but not in those that were fed. These changes were associated with an increase in the level of ^{14}C covalently bound in the liver following exposure to [^{14}C]-vinylidene chloride (section 6.1.5). Hepatotoxic effects were not noted in either fed or fasted rats exposed to 40 mg vinylidene chloride/m^3 (10 ppm). In a more recent study, inhalation of vinylidene chloride produced acute nephrotoxicity (which was not associated with calcium oxalate formation) in male Sprague-Dawley rats [90]. Twenty-four hours after a 4-h exposure to 1000 mg vinylidene chloride/m^3 (250 ppm) or more, kidney/body weight ratios, serum urea nitrogen, and creatinine levels were significantly increased. This was associated with moderate cellular swelling in the renal cortex (800 mg/m^3 (200 ppm)) and severe tubular necrosis (>1200 mg/m^3 (>300 ppm)). Aroclor-1254 and phenobarbital pretreatment antagonized renal toxicity.

1.1.2 Mice

A marked individual variation in the lethal concentration of vinylidene chloride (ranging from 500 to 10 000 mg/m^3; 125 to 2500 ppm) was noted by Lazarev [116].

In the study by Short et al. [204], the toxicity of inhaled vinylidene chloride was investigated in CD-1 mice. The 1- and 2-day LC$_{50}$ values for groups of 10 mice were approximately 400 mg/m^3 (100 ppm) (males and females) and 140 mg/m^3 (35 ppm) (males), respectively. These values are considerably lower than those reported for rats and, in contrast to the data on mice, no deaths were seen in male rats exposed to 240 mg vinylidene chloride/m^3 (60 ppm). In addition, up to 240 mg vinylidene chloride/m^3 (60 ppm) produced a dose-dependent histopathological change in mouse liver and an increase in both serum glutamic oxaloacetic transaminase and serum glutamic pyruvic transaminase. The serum enzymes were also elevated in male rats but not to the same extent and only with a longer exposure period. Mice exposed for 1 day to 60 mg vinylidene chloride/m^3 (15 ppm) showed hepatocellular degeneration and increased mitotic figures of hepatocytes together with severe kidney tubular nephrosis. At 120 mg/m^3 (30 ppm), midzonal hepatic necrosis was also seen, the severity of which was increased at 240 mg/m^3 (60 ppm). In contrast, rats exposed to 240 mg/m^3 (60 ppm) for 1 day showed only mild hepatic centrilobular degeneration and/or necrosis and mild bile-duct hyperplasia. The inhibition of these toxic effects and of covalent binding of [^{14}C]-vinylidene chloride-derived radioactivity in the mouse liver and kidney by disulfiram was described. The mechanism of this protection was not established but may be via modulation of metabolism.

The studies of Zeller et al. [250] on NMRI mice showed that, as with rats, males were more susceptible than females (Table 7) and that fasting potentiated lethality. Symptoms included apathy, narcosis, dyspnoea, and immobility. Post-mortem examination of mice dying from vinylidene chloride exposure particularly showed acute emphysema and congestion of lungs.

The effects of vinylidene chloride on DNA following acute inhalation (40 or 200 mg/m^3 (10 or 50 ppm) for 6 h) have been studied in male CD-1 mice as well as Sprague-Dawley rats [186]. These exposures gave rise to tissue damage (nephrosis, increased mitotic figures, and regeneration) and increased DNA semiconservative replication (25-fold) in mouse kidney, but not in mouse liver. In contrast, DNA semiconservative replication in rat kidney was increased only 2.2 fold and was slightly decreased in rat liver following exposure to 40 mg/m^3 (10 ppm). DNA repair and DNA alkylation in these organs were minimal in both rats and mice (section 8.5.1). In the light of these minimal effects, the authors suggested that the carcinogenicity of vinylidene chloride in the mouse kidney (section 8.7.1) might be via an epigenetic mechanism.

8.1.1.3 Other animal species

Effects of vinylidene chloride on the respiratory system have also been reported in cats, rabbits, and guinea-pigs [192]. Pulmonary irritation and lung oedema, haemorrhage, and pneumonia were seen following exposure to vinylidene chloride at 2000 or 6000 mg/m^3 (500 or 1500 ppm) (cats) and 5000 or 8000 mg/m^3 (1250 or 2000 ppm) (guinea-pigs) for 2 h. Exposure to concentrations ranging from 500 to 2000 mg/m^3 (125 to 500 ppm) for 40 min inhibited spinal reflexes in rabbits. This species survived after exposure for 40 min to a concentration of 30 000 mg/m^3 (7500 ppm). Klimisch & Freisberg [108, 109] studied the inhalation toxicity of vinylidene chloride in fed and fasted Chinese striped hamsters. The LC$_{50}$ values are given in Table 7. As with rats and mice, males were more susceptible to lethality than females, and fasting potentiated the toxicity markedly. Hamsters that died showed acute dilation and passive hyperaemia of the heart, congested lungs, and lobulation of the liver.

8.1.2 Oral

As with inhalation, the principal organs affected by oral administration of vinylidene chloride are the liver, kidneys, and lungs.

The LD$_{50}$ values for orally administered vinylidene chloride in rats and mice are shown in Table 7. It can again be seen that mice are more susceptible than rats, but few sex differences in response are observed following administration of vinylidene chloride by gavage.

1.2.1 Rats

Hepatic damage produced by intubation of 400 mg vinylidene chloride/kg to fasted rats was indicated by elevation of serum alanine α-ketoglutarate transaminase activity within 4 h [94]. The level of glucose-6-phosphatase activity was reduced in the liver at 8 h, but not after 4 h, suggesting (in line with the above discussion) that initial toxicity was not associated with the endoplasmic reticulum membrane. Treatment of rats with a relatively high dose of 12.5 mmol vinylidene chloride/kg did not lead to elevation of malondialdehyde or conjugated dienes in incubated liver homogenates taken 1 h after dosing. This contrasts with the effect of a hepatotoxic dose of carbon tetrachloride and suggests that lipid peroxidation is not involved in the hepatotoxicity of vinylidene chloride.

Jenkins et al. [100] also reported, that pretreatment of rats with the microsomal enzyme-inducing agent phenobarbital offered protection against the hepatotoxic effects of orally administered vinylidene chloride. The acute 24-h toxicity of vinylidene chloride was enhanced 18-fold by adrenalectomy, suggesting that the adrenals were involved in protection against lethal effects. The mechanisms of protection were not understood.

The effects of induction and inhibition of microsomal enzymes in fasted male Holtzman rats were studied in more detail by Andersen et al. [4]. Pretreatment of rats with phenobarbital markedly reduced the lethality of a 100 mg/kg oral dose of vinylidene chloride in immature rats (140 g), but not in large adult (331 g) rats.

These results suggest that a microsomal detoxification system, inducible in immature rats, was operative. This is supported by the finding that the cytochrome P-450 inhibitor SKF-525A exacerbated the lethal effects of a dose of vinylidene chloride of 200 mg/kg in rats (260–270 g) but did not have any effect on mortality in immature (80–100 g) 2,3-epoxy-propan-1-ol, rats. One of a range of epoxides that exacerbate the toxicity of orally administered vinylidene chloride, which is particularly potent, was a relatively poor substrate for glutathione-S-transferase and styrene oxide hydrolase. Thus 2,3-epoxypropan-1-ol, rather than inhibiting the protective effects of epoxide hydrolase or glutathione conjugation (section 6.1.4) appeared to inhibit a further (uncharacterized) detoxification pathway [3]. The role of a further microsomal enzyme system in the production of a toxic intermediate was indicated by the protective effects of pretreatment of rats of all sizes with pyrazole, 3-aminotriazole, and carbon tetrachloride against the lethality of an oral dose of 200 mg/kg [4].

Andersen & Jenkins [2] noted that female Holtzman HOT:(SD)BR rats were much less susceptible to the hepatotoxic effect than male rats, the threshold oral dose for the elevation of plasma transaminase activity being approximately 100 mg/kg in the females. When mature, male rats were given 400 mg vinylidene chloride/kg, levels of plasma-aspartate transaminase were 4–5 times greater in 18-h fasted rats than in control rats. The effects of fasting are thought to be due to glutathione depletion (section 6.1.5). Chieco et al. [28] studied hepatotoxicity in fasted male Sprague-Dawley rats given vinylidene chloride as an oral dose in mineral oil. Two hours after dosing with 200 mg vinylidene chloride/kg or 6 h after a lower dose of 50 mg/kg, early damage to plasma and mitochondrial membranes was indicated by raised hepatic sodium levels and decreased central area histochemical staining of bile canaliculi membrane Mg^{2+}-ATPase, outer membrane mitochondrial monoamine oxidase, and inner membrane mitochondrial succinate dehydrogenase and cytochrome oxidase. The extent of injury (indicated by raised serum transaminase activity and decreased histochemical staining of membrane components) increased with time after dosing or with increased dose. Four and 6 h after administration of a 200 mg/kg dose, necrosis occurred around the central vein of the liver. There were no histochemical alterations in the kidneys at 6 h. The same investigators [27] noted that this treatment produced increased plasma-haemoglobin levels and granular "haem" casts in the loop of Henlé. No pathological changes were seen in the heart, lungs, spleen, adrenals, or duodenum. Hepatic damage was more severe with Tween 80 used as a dose vehicle than with corn oil or mineral oil, reflecting a relatively high rate of absorption when administered in Tween 80 (section 6.1.1.2).

Eight hours after oral administration of 40 mg vinylidene chloride/kg body weight to rats, centrilobular hepatocytes showed a dilated endoplasmic reticulum and swollen mitochondria and perinuclear cisternae. The nucleosplasm was homogeneous suggesting chromatinolysis [5].

In unanaesthetized, freely moving fed and fasted Sprague-Dawley male rats [148], at least a 2-fold increase in inulin excretion was observed within 2 h of oral administration of 200 mg vinylidene chloride/kg. Bile flow decreased in treated rats (up to 40% and 65% in the fed and fasted rats, respectively). Thus, vinylidene chloride alters hepatobiliary permeability and causes cholestasis.

Kanz & Reynolds [105] investigated the occurrence of morphological changes in the liver in relation to time after oral administration of vinylidene chloride (25, 50, or 100 mg/kg in mineral oil) (see also Kanz et al. [106], reported in section 8.1.1.1). One, 2, or 3 h after administration to fasted male Sprague-Dawley rats, the liver was examined microscopically following *in situ* perfusion fixation. Dilation of the bile canaliculi with an increase in the number of microvilli or membrane fragments in canaliculi was seen with the formation of canalicular diverticuli in centrilobular hepatocytes within 1–2 h. Subsequently, microvilli on the sinusoidal surfaces were lost, and cytoplasmic vacuolation occurred. These early changes were seen without morphological alteration of the endoplasmic reticulum or mitochondria. Not until 4–6 h after an oral dose of 200 mg vinylidene chloride/kg was a decrease seen in the activity of enzymes in the sinusoidal plasma, mitochondrial matrix, endoplasmic reticulum, lysosomes and cytosol, and then only in regions of gross injury. At 2 h, scattered hepatocytes showed nuclear and cell surface anomalies that were characteristic of apoptosis [190].

In agreement with the findings of Reynolds et al. [189] in inhalation studies (section 8.1.1.1), Moslen & Reynolds [147] found that loss of activity of microsomal cytochrome P-450 was not an early event in the toxicity of vinylidene chloride (200 mg/kg) orally administered to fasted male Sprague-Dawley rats. Cytochrome P-450 deactivation was concomitant with an elevation in the activities of serum glutamate oxalacetate transaminase and serum glutamate pyruvate transaminase and did not occur until between 2 and 3 h after administration of vinylidene chloride. These effects were preceded by a marked inhibition (within 1 h) of the activity of glutathione-S-transferase towards dichloronitrobenzene, chlorodinitrobenzene, and 1,2-epoxy-3-(p-nitrophenoxy)-propane (but not towards ethacrynic acid) and a concomitant reduction of hepatic glutathione levels. A correlation was found between the dose-dependency of inhibition of glutathione-S-transferase activity and of cytotoxicity. Thus, both glutathione depletion and inhibition of specific glutathione-S-transferase(s) precede toxicity.

Simultaneous treatment of 8 male Wistar rats with ethanol (4.8 g/kg, oral) protected against the hepatotoxicity of vinylidene chloride (0.125 g/kg, oral) as measured by the elevation of the activities of serum aminotransferases and sorbitol dehydrogenase [208]. Conversely, pretreatment of rats with ethanol (5% in drinking-water for 7 days) exacerbated the hepatotoxicity of orally administered vinylidene chloride (0.125 or 0.2 g/kg). Dithiocarb or (+)-catechin (0.2 g/kg) administered simultaneously with vinylidene chloride also reduced vinylidene chloride-induced hepatotoxicity. Evidence was provided that the simultaneous treatment with ethanol and dithiocarb may lead to depression of the metabolism of vinylidene chloride. It was postulated that (+)-catechin might act as a scavenger of reactive intermediate(s), which may also be the mechanism of protection afforded by (+)-cyanidanol-3 [207].

Acetone is another agent that modifies the hepatotoxicity of orally administered vinylidene chloride [75]. Administration of 5 or 10 mmol acetone/kg orally to male Sprague-Dawley rats potentiated liver injury (elevated plasma glutamic pyruvic transaminase and ornithine carbamyl transferase activity and liver total bilirubin content) caused by a single oral dose of 50 mg vinylidene chloride/kg. However, acetone given at 1, 15, or 30 mmol/kg, did not potentiate hepatotoxicity. The biphasic effect of acetone could not be explained but was considered by the authors to be related to dose-dependent changes in more than one biotransformation process.

A further effect of vinylidene chloride was the prolongation of barbiturate sleeping times [92]. Two to 4 h after an oral dose of 400 mg vinylidene chloride/kg to male Holtzman rats, the pentobarbital sleeping time was elevated (136% of control), (prior to hepatotoxicity as indicated by loss of glucose-6-phosphatase activity). Both hexobarbital and pentobarbital sleeping times were elevated at 17-22 h, concomitant with hepatic injury. The early effects on pentobarbital sleeping times were due, not to decreased metabolism of the barbiturate, but to an elevation of its concentration in serum through altered absorption or distribution.

Kidney toxicity was studied by Jenkins & Andersen [99] in NMRI:0(SD), Sprague-Dawley-derived rats. Within 24 h of oral administration of 400 mg vinylidene chloride/kg, fasted male rats showed raised levels of plasma urea nitrogen and creatinine. Within 48 h, tubular dilation was observed with necrosis and vacuolation of tubular epithelium. Some tubules contained a blue-black amorphous material. These histopathological effects were preceded by inflammation in some animals. Elevation of plasma urea nitrogen and creatinine was not observed in fed rats with identical treatment and was less evident in fasted females than in males. However, the histopathological effects were no less severe in the female rats. The time-course for the nephrotoxic response (maximum at 48 h) in male and female fasted rats was slightly preceded by hepatotoxicity as indicated by the appearance in the plasma of aspartate transaminase, alanine transaminase lactate dehydrogenase, and sorbitol dehydrogenase (maximum at 8–24 h). This finding is in agreement with that reported above [28].

8.1.2.2 Mice

Orally administered vinylidene chloride also caused pulmonary injury in male C57B1/6 mice [52]. Following administration of 100 mg/kg, peribronchial and perivascular oedema were seen in the lungs. Histopathology revealed dilation of Clara cell cisternae and degeneration of the endoplasmic reticulum. A 200 mg/kg dose caused severe necrosis of ciliated and Clara cells and exfoliation of the bronchial lining within 6 h. Both doses caused concurrent hepatotoxicity as evidenced by raised levels of serum glutamic oxalacetic transaminase and glutamic pyruvic transaminase. By 24 h, pulmonary oedema, haemorrhage, and focal atelectasis were also observed in association with hypoxia. Recovery was seen within 7 days. Following a higher dose of 200 mg/kg, injury was seen to be followed by cellular proliferation as indicated by incorporation of a pulse of [^{3}H]-thymidine into total pulmonary DNA [53]. Proliferative activity reached a peak between 3 and 5 days after treatment with vinylidene chloride. The majority of the ^{3}H was incorporated into non-ciliated bronchiolar epithelial cells.

8.1.3 Other routes

8.1.3.1 Intraperitoneal

When given by intraperitoneal (ip) injection to male ddY strain mice at a dose level of 120 mg/kg (0.1 ml/kg), vinylidene chloride produced hypothermia within 30 min and severe renal damage at 24 h (as shown by elevated plasma urea nitrogen and kidney calcium levels) [143]. Renal tubular necrosis was much more severe than hepatic damage. Pretreatment of mice with diethyldithiocarbamate or carbon disulfide protected against renal and hepatic toxicity, possibly via an inhibitory effect on metabolic activation. Vinylidene chloride at 605 mg/kg (0.5 ml/kg, ip) caused liver damage in male Sprague-Dawley rats as evidenced by raised serum glutamate pyruvate transaminase and increased bile duct pancreatic fluid flow at 24 h [70]. Hepatic microsomal glucose-6-phosphatase and ATP-dependent calcium pump were both inhibited 24 h after intraperitoneal administration of vinylidene chloride (1 mg/kg) to male Sprague-Dawley rats [145]. The level of conjugated dienes in microsomes obtained 2 h after vinylidene chloride injection was not significantly different from that measured in control rat microsomes, suggesting that the toxic effects were not mediated by lipid peroxidation.

The results of Siegers et al. [209] also suggest that lipid peroxidation is not a mechanism involved in the early stages of vinylidene chloride hepatotoxicity. Up to 2 h after an intraperitoneal injection of 0.5 g vinylidene chloride/kg to male Wistar rats, ethane exhalation was only slightly higher than the control levels and was not affected by hypoxia.

As was observed in the short-term inhalation studies on vinylidene chloride (section 8.2.1), the compound was found to induce cytochrome P-450 activity following a single administration to C57B1/6N mice by intraperitoneal injection. Over the range of 50–150 mg/kg, a dose-dependent induction of microsomal 7-ethoxyresorufin and 7-ethoxycoumarin O-deethylation (but not total cytochrome P-450 content or benzo(a)pyrene hydroxylase) was found in the kidney [112].

Male C57BL/6J mice given 125 mg vinylidene chloride/kg (ip) developed extensive necrosis of the Clara cells in the lung within 24 h, but no necrosis was observed in the liver or kidney at this time. The loss of Clara cells was associated with a significant decrease in pulmonary cytochrome P-450 content and activity [113]. The susceptibility of the Clara cells was considered to be due to activation of vinylidene chloride by cytochrome P-450 in these cells. This conclusion was also reached by Forkert et al. [55] who showed that covalent binding of vinylidene chloride products to cellular macromolecules in the lung accompanied lung toxicity in CD-1 mice given an identical dose to that given in the study described above (section 6.1.5). Degenerative changes occurred in Clara cells as early as 1 h following treatment with vinylidene chloride and were characterized by mitochondrial swelling and aggregation of chromatin against the nuclear membrane. Cell death was apparent at 2 h and, by 24 h, the majority of Clara cells were exfoliated [56]. However, these authors concluded that there was a lack of correlation between the extent of covalent binding and either lung or liver toxicity [55].

8.1.3.2 Eyes and skin

Little information is available on the effects of vinylidene chloride on the eyes and skin.

It is moderately irritating to the eyes of rabbits causing transient corneal injury and is also a skin irritant in the rabbit [222]. Rylova, [192] reported that vinylidene chloride was an irritant for the eyes of rats, mice, guinea-pigs, and cats.

Transient redness was observed following application to shaved rabbit skin. The stabilizer (p-methoxyphenol) in vinylidene chloride preparations may contribute to irritation.

8.1.4 Summary of acute toxicity

Vinylidene chloride may cause irritation of the skin and eye, depression of the central nervous system, and acute toxic effects on the heart, lung, liver, and kidney. The variation in estimations of the acute LC_{50} for vinylidene chloride is considerable. This can be explained partially by inaccuracies that arise because of a non-linear concentration- mortality relationship. Generally, mice are more susceptible than rats and males are more susceptible than females. The toxic effects are dependent on cytochrome P-450 activity (which may also be involved in detoxification) and can be exacerbated by glutathione depletion. Hepatotoxicity may be enhanced by ethanol and thyroxine, inhibited by dithiocarb and (+)-catechin, and modulated by acetone.

8.2 Short-Term Exposures

8.2.1 Inhalation

In the study by Prendergast et al. [173], groups of various animal species were continuously or repeatedly exposed to vinylidene chloride through inhalation for 90 days. The results are shown in Table 8. In survivors of continuous exposure at a concentration of 101 mg/m^3 or less, no histopathological changes could be attributed

Table 8. Mortality of animals exposed to vinylidene chloride by inhalation[a]

Concentration of vinylidene chloride (mg/m^3)	Extent of exposure[c]	Mortality ratio[b]				
		Rat (Long Evans or Sprague-Dawley)	Guinea-pig (Hartley)	Rabbit (New Zealand White)	Beagle dog	Squirrel monkey
395 ± 32	A	0/15	0/15	0/3	0/2	0/3
189 ± 6.2	B	0/15	7/15	-	0/2	3/9
101 ± 4.4	B	0/15	3/15	0/3	0/2	2/3
61 ± 5.7	B	0/15	3/15	-	0/2	0/9
20 ± 2.1	B	2/45	2/45	-	0/6	1/21
no treatment	B	7/304	2/314	2/48	0/34	1/57

[a] From: Prendergast et al. [173].
[b] Mortality ratio shows the number of animals that died divided by the number with which the study commenced.
[c] A = 30 exposures, 8 h/day, 5 days/week.
B = continuous 90-day exposure.

to vinylidene chloride. At 189 mg/m^3, livers from surviving dogs, monkeys, and rats showed morphological changes consisting of fatty metamorphosis, focal necrosis, haemosiderin deposition, lymphocytic infiltration, bile-duct proliferation, fibrosis, and pseudolobule formation, particularly in dogs. All rats displayed nuclear hypertrophy of the kidney tubular epithelium. Non-specific inflammatory changes were seen in the lungs of a majority of the animals. Liver alkaline phosphatase activity and serum glutamic-pyruvic transaminase activity were measured in rats and guinea-pigs and found to be elevated. Dogs, monkeys, and rats showed reduced weight gain. The repeated exposures are considered to be more relevant to human occupational exposure. Gross examination of survivors showed a high incidence of lung congestion in rabbits, monkeys, rats, and guinea-pigs. Some fatty infiltration and several cases of focal and sub-massive necrosis were observed in guinea-pig liver sections.

Shortly after this study, Gage [57] investigated the toxicity of vinylidene chloride in Alderley Park rats. In this case, groups of 4 male and 4 female rats were exposed to 2000 mg vinylidene chloride/m^3 (500 ppm) for 6 h per day over a period of 20 days. Nose irritation and retarded weight gain were observed, and, at autopsy, liver cell degeneration was detected by histology. At 800 mg/m^3 (200 ppm) (4 male and 4 female rats), slight nose irritation was seen, but the organs were normal on autopsy.

Inhalation studies [152, 176] demonstrated minimal recoverable liver cell cytoplasmic vacuolation in Sprague-Dawley rats (20 animals per sex) after 90 days exposure for 6 h per day, 5 days/week, to vinylidene chloride at 100 or 300 mg/m^3 (25 or 75 ppm). At both dose levels, body weight, haematology, urinalyses, blood urea nitrogen, serum alkaline phosphatase and glutamic pyruvic transaminase activities, gross pathology, organ weights, kidneys, heart, testes, and brain were normal.

Maltoni & Patella [138] noted a greater toxicity in rats than that reported by Gage [57]. The effects of 4 h exposure, 4–5 days per week, for 28 days, were studied in Sprague-Dawley rats and Swiss mice (40–800 mg/m^3 (10–200 ppm)), Balb/c, C3H, and C57B1 mice (600–800 mg/m^3 (150–200 ppm)), and Chinese hamsters (100 mg/m^3 (25 ppm) only). The exposure periods were reduced at or above 200 mg/m^3 (50 ppm) in mice because of severe acute toxicity, and the 800 mg/m^3 (200 ppm) treatment of rats was reduced to 600 mg/m^3 (150 ppm) after 2 days because of toxic effects. A minimum of 30 animals was used in all groups exposed to vinylidene chloride.

The weight of animals, clinical signs of toxicity, mortality, and histopathological changes were monitored at, or up to, 28 days, except in the case of mice exposed to 400–800 mg/m^3 (100–200 ppm), when the observation period was 9 days. Histopathological studies indicated that the liver and kidneys were the major target organs. The toxicity varied with animal species and strain, susceptibility being in the following order: Swiss mice > Balb/c mice > C3H mice > C57B1 mice > rats. In general, females were less responsive than males, with the exception of female C3H mice, which were more susceptible than the females of the other strains tested. An association between the occurrence of acute toxicity and the reported carcinogenicity in the Swiss mouse was noted (section 8.7.4). Another comparison study also indicated marked strain and sex differences in the response of mice to vinylidene chloride [153]. The mice (10 males and 10 females per dose level) were exposed to 220, 400, or 800 mg vinylidene chloride/m^3 (55, 100, or 200 ppm) for 6 h/day, 5 days/week, for a total of 10 exposures. Only at 800 mg/m^3 (200 ppm) were exposure-related deaths observed and the rates of mortality were greater in the males than in the females in Ha (ICR), CD-1 and CF-W mice, but no sex-related differences in mortality were observed in B$_6$C$_3$F mice. Gross and histopathological examinations indicated that nephrotoxicity accounted for mortality in the male mice, but this was not the case in female mice. Hepatotoxicity was considered to be the cause of death in Ha (ICR) and B$_6$C$_3$F$_1$ mice. The greatest sensitivity to renal toxicity was seen in male CF-W mice (a strain derived from the Swiss-Webster strain, believed to be genetically comparable to Maltoni's Swiss mouse).

The greater susceptibility to vinylidene chloride of mice compared with rats was also shown by Short et al. [204], agreeing with the findings from acute single exposures (section 8.1). After 2 days exposure to 240 mg/m^3 (60 ppm), 8/10 and 0/10 deaths were recorded in male CD-1 mice and male CD rats, respectively. No mice survived a longer period of exposure at 240 mg/m^3 (60 ppm). Serum glutamic oxaloacetic transaminase and glutamic pyruvic transaminase levels were raised in both rats and mice, but more so in the latter. Severe hepatotoxicity and nephrotoxicity were observed in mice at autopsy.

A comparative study on the short-term toxicity of vinylidene chloride in male Sprague-Dawley rats and in both sexes of Swiss-Webster mice was reported by Oesch et al. [156]. Animals (minimum of 10 per group) were exposed to an atmosphere containing vinylidene chloride at 40 or 200 mg/m^3 (10 or 50 ppm) (mice) or 800 mg/m^3 (200 ppm) (rats) for 6 h, on 1, 3, or 8 days, and killed one day after the last treatment. The majority of male mice exposed to 200 mg/m^3 (50 ppm) for 8 days did not survive. However, female mice survived this treatment as did rats exposed to 800 mg/m^3

(200 ppm). Various changes in the activities of monooxygenase, epoxide hydrolase, and glutathione transferase enzymes occurred in animals treated with vinylidene chloride. The enzyme changes could contribute to the relative susceptibility of the animals, according to the balance of activating and detoxifying activity. In particular, cytosolic glutathione transferase activity towards the substrate 2,4-dinitrochlorobenzene was decreased in the kidneys of male mice (an organ susceptible to carcinogenicity (section 8.7.1)), but not in the kidney of rats or female mice or in the liver of either of these species (where activity was either unchanged or enhanced).

A study on rabbits has also been reported by Lazarev [116]. Bronchitis, degenerative changes in the liver and kidney, and an increase in the rate of proliferation of lymphoid tissue in the spleen were observed in animals exposed to concentrations of 500–2000 mg vinylidene chloride/m^3 (125–500 ppm) for 3 h/day over a period of 4 months.

In summary, a number of studies have indicated the particular susceptibility of the male Swiss mouse to kidney toxicity. This strain, sex, and species selectivity has important implications regarding the specificity of the carcinogenic action of vinylidene chloride (section 8.7.4).

8.2.2 Oral

In a 90-day study, vinylidene chloride was incorporated in the drinking-water of male and female Sprague-Dawley rats at nominal concentrations of 0, 60, 100 or 200 mg/litre [152,176]. Even at the highest concentrations administered (equivalent to 19–26 mg/kg body weight daily), only minimal, reversible liver cytoplasmic vacuolation was observed, with no abnormalities in any of the other parameters investigated (section 8.2.1). Maltoni & Patella [138] also noted a lack of lethality and clinical signs of toxicity in Sprague-Dawley rats (50 of each sex) orally dosed by gavage with 0, 0.5, 5, 10, or 20 mg vinylidene chloride/kg for 28 consecutive days. Four female and 4 male beagle dogs were given 6.25, 12.5, or 25 mg vinylidene chloride/kg in peanut oil incorporated in gelatin capsules, daily for 97 days [177]. No significant differences were seen between these animals and controls with respect to appearance and demeanor, mortality, body weight, food consumption, haematology, urinalysis, clinical chemistry, and organ weights. There was also no depletion in hepatic non-protein sulfhydryl levels in the liver or kidneys.

Some evidence for hepatotoxicity was provided by Siegers et al. [208] using higher levels of orally administered vinylidene chloride. Male Wistar rats were given 0.125 g vinylidene chloride/kg in olive oil, by gavage, twice weekly for 2 weeks, followed by a similar treatment at 0.2 g/kg for 2 weeks. Hepatotoxicity was evidenced by mild increases in serum sorbitol dehydrogenase and aminotransferases. Ethanol co-treatment (5% in drinking-water) with the 0.2 g/kg dose of vinylidene chloride enhanced toxicity leading to 6 deaths out of 10 animals. Simultaneous application of dithiocarb or (+)-catechin with vinylidene chloride led to total protection against lethal effects. The effects of these agents have been discussed elsewhere (section 8.1.2.1).

8.3 Long-Term Exposure

A number of studies described in this section are also discussed in section 8.7 in relation to carcinogenicity.

8.3.1 Inhalation

Sprague-Dawley rats, 84–86 of each sex, 6–7 weeks of age at the start of the study, were exposed to vinylidene chloride vapour at 0, 40, or 160 mg/m^3 (0, 10, or 40 ppm) for, 6 h/day, 5 days/week, for 5 weeks, after which the levels of vinylidene chloride were changed to 0, 100, and 300 mg/m^3 (0, 25, and 75 ppm) [178,179,180]. After exposure for a total of 18 months, the rats were observed for a further 6 months. Additional animals were used for interim kills at 1, 6, and 12 months. No clinical signs of toxicity were seen in the exposed groups. Mean body weight gain was reduced at both dose levels during the period of 8–13 months in males, but was not reduced in females. Mortality in exposed groups was only slightly higher than that in the controls (not different at the 40–100 mg/m^3 (10–25 ppm) dose levels in males) and only in the latter part of the study. Histopathological studies indicated increased cytoplasmic vacuolation in the livers of exposed animals at 6 and 12 months of exposure. During the 6-month postexposure period of the study, the hepatic changes were no longer discernible, indicating reversibility.

There was also evidence of liver damage in CD-1 mice and CD rats (groups of 36 males and 36 females) exposed to 220 mg vinylidene chloride/m^3 (55 ppm) (6 h/day, 5 days/week); the animals were about 2 months old at the start of the study. Four animals of each species and sex were killed for examination after 1, 2, 3, 6, and 9 months of treatment. The remaining animals were killed at 12 months [118]. Groups of 100 animals were used as controls. No effects were seen regarding haematology, clinical blood chemistry, pulmonary macrophage count, cytogenic analysis of bone marrow, X-ray examination of extremities, serum α-fetoprotein, collagen content of liver, and lung and serum or urinary aminolevulinic acid (ALA) (collagen and ALA were not measured in the mice). However, mice exposed to vinylidene chloride for 6–12 months had enlarged and basophilic hepatocytes with enlarged nuclei, focal degeneration, and necrosis. A mild to markedly severe focal disseminated vacuolization of the liver was seen in the treated rats.

A similar long-term toxicity study was carried out by Hong et al. [79] on male and female CD-1 mice and CD rats exposed to 220 mg vinylidene chloride /m^3 (55 ppm) or filtered air (controls), for 6 h/day, 5 days/week. The numbers of rats used per sex group were 4, 8, 8, and 14–16, and these were exposed for 1, 3, 6, and 10 months, respectively. Mice (8, 8, and 12 animals per sex group) were exposed for 1, 3, and 6 months, respectively. Animals were aged 2 months at the start of the study and were observed for 12 months after treatment. No histopathological changes were observed as a result of these treatments with vinylidene chloride. A total of 11/24 mice exposed for 6 months died or were terminated in a moribund condition (compared with 11/56 controls). Only 3 rats died following exposure for 6 months or less (20/30 rats died in the group exposed for 10 months compared with 13/32 controls).

Long-term inhalation toxicity was also studied in rats, mice, and hamsters by Maltoni et al. [141]. Groups of male and female Sprague-Dawley rats (60 of each) were exposed to 40, 100, 200, 400, 600, or 800 mg vinylidene chloride/m^3 (10, 25, 50, 100, 150, or 200 ppm), for 4 h/day, 4–5 days/week, for 52 weeks. Unexposed control groups consisted of 100 rats of each sex. The rats were 16 weeks old at the start of the study. At spontaneous death, hepatocyte vacuolization, cloudy swelling, fatty degeneration, necrobiosis, and necrosis were more frequent (57.6%) in rats exposed to 800–600 mg/m^3 (200–150 ppm) than in control animals (20.5%). The highest tolerable dose for long-term exposure in rats was 600 mg/m^3 (150 ppm). In Swiss mice (aged either 9 or 16 weeks at the start of the study) exposed to 40 or 100 mg vinylidene chloride/m^3 (10 or 25 ppm) for the same exposure periods (minimum of 30 mice per sex per dose level), changes were seen in the liver and kidneys that were compatible with changes seen in long-term studies on control animals. However, a higher incidence of regressive or phlogistic changes was seen in the kidneys with renal adenocarcinoma (section 8.7.1) at 100 mg/m^3 (25 ppm). A high mortality was seen at 200 mg/m^3 (50 ppm). Those that survived only 4 exposures had hepatic fibrosis, which was considered to be due to repair of necrosis. Chinese hamsters (30 male and 30 female) exposed to a concentration of 100 mg vinylidene chloride/m^3 (25 ppm) for periods identical to those given above for rats and mice, showed no signs of altered histology compared with controls (18 male and 17 female) at spontaneous death.

Thus, the most significant observation on toxicity from long-term inhalation studies is that of dose-dependent kidney damage in male Swiss mice at dose levels that were not nephrotoxic in female mice or in other species tested. The findings have important implications in the light of similar tissue, sex, and species specificities in carcinogenicity (section 8.7.1).

8.3.2 Oral

The long-term oral toxicity of vinylidene chloride was investigated by Maltoni et al. [141] in Sprague-Dawley rats at 0.5, 5, 10, or 20 mg/kg (given once daily by stomach tube, 4–5 days/week, for 52 weeks). Animals were aged 9 or 10 weeks at the start of the study. Fifty animals of each sex were used per dose group with 100 controls (except for the 0.5 mg/kg group where there were 160 controls). No signs of toxicity were reported from a complete autopsy after 147 weeks (or 136 weeks, 0.5 mg/kg) except that "hepatocyte vacuolization, cloudy swelling, fatty degeneration, necrobiosis, and necrosis were found in some animals in treated as well as in control groups".

In a separate study, 48 Sprague-Dawley rats of each sex (aged 6–7 weeks at the start of the study) were given vinylidene chloride in the drinking-water at the following dose levels for 2 years: 7, 10, or 20 mg/kg body weight for males and 9, 14, or 30 mg/kg for females (nominally 50, 100, and 200 mg/litre drinking-water). Eighty rats per sex were dosed as control groups without vinylidene chloride treatment [177, 179, 180]. Various parameters were monitored, as indicated for the 90-day study (section 8.2.1). Slightly increased cytoplasmic vacuolation of hepatocytes and hepatocellular fatty change were the only evidence of toxicity and occurred at all dose levels in the females, but only at 20 mg/kg body weight (200 mg/litre drinking-water) in the males.

A US National Toxicology Programme study [154] indicated chronic renal inflammation in male and female F344/N rats (50 per group) given 5 mg vinylidene chloride/kg in corn oil, by gavage, 5 times/week, for 104 weeks. At 1 mg/kg, no renal toxicity was observed. In all treated rats, the clinical signs and histopathology of other organs were the same as in control rats. This group also studied long-term oral toxicity in male and female $B_6C_3F_1/N$ mice (50 per group) administered 2 or 10 mg/kg in corn oil. At 10 mg/kg, necrosis of the liver was evident in male but not in female mice, but the reverse was true at the 2 mg/kg dose level. However, the sponsors found defects in the conduct of the study and it could not be satisfactorily evaluated.

Ponomarkov & Tomatis [172] gave rats an oral dose of vinylidene chloride (50 mg/kg) weekly for the life span of the animal following an initial *in utero* exposure (section 8.7.2 for details). Rats that died up to 30 weeks after the start of oral dosing (7/89 males and 7/90 females) showed congestion of the lungs and kidneys. At up to 80–90 weeks, haemorrhages and multiple lobular necrosis of the liver were observed. The numbers of animals that survived for 90 weeks were 71/89 (males) and 75/90 (females) compared with 49/50 and 47/53 male and female controls, respectively. Some of the treated survivors of 90 weeks showed degenerative lesions of liver parenchymal cells.

8.4 Toxicity in vitro

As revealed in in vivo studies ([145] section 8.1.3.1), in vitro studies with rat liver microsomes showed that calcium pump activity was inhibited in a dose-dependent manner by vinylidene chloride in the presence of NADPH. Malonic dialdehyde production (a consequence of lipid peroxidation) was not associated with inhibition of the calcium pump [182].

These findings stimulated Long & Moore [126] to test whether vinylidene chloride treatment of hepatocytes could raise cytosolic Ca^{2+} concentrations. Isolated hepatocytes from Sprague-Dawley rats were exposed to vinylidene chloride (4 mmol/litre). Within 5 min, the concentration of Ca^{2+} (estimated from the activity of glycogen phosphorylase a) was raised to 0.3 μmol/litre compared with 0.04 μmol/litre in vehicle-treated controls. In separate studies, the concentration of Ca^{2+} was measured in hepatocytes loaded with quin 2 (a sensitive fluorescent indicator of cytoplasmic concentrations of ionized calcium). Within 20 seconds of addition of vinylidene chloride at 4 mmol/litre, Ca^{2+} levels were increased from 0.26 ± 0.05 μmol/litre to 0.59 ± 0.06 μmol/litre. Disruption of intracellular Ca^{2+} homeostasis may prove to be a mechanism that can contribute to vinylidene chloride hepatotoxicity.

8.5 Mutagenicity and Other Genotoxicity Assays

8.5.1 Interaction with DNA

The fact that a number of metabolites of vinylidene chloride are reactive and covalently bind to cellular macromolecules and the nucleophile glutathione has already been discussed in section 6.1.5. The specific covalent interaction with DNA has been little studied. As reported in section 8.1.1.2, DNA binding in vivo in rats and mice exposed to [^{14}C]-vinylidene chloride at 40 mg/m^3 (10 ppm) (rats) and 40 or 200 mg/m^3 (10 or 50 ppm) (mice) for 6 h was minimal, though DNA adducts were evident from the covalently bound radiolabel [186]. Adduct formation was greater in mice than in rats and greater in the kidneys than in the liver. Binding was dose dependent in the kidneys of mice (equivalent to 30 adducts/10^6 nucleotides at 200 mg vinylidene chloride/m^3 (50 ppm) and 11 adducts/10^6 nucleotides at 40 mg/m^3 (10 ppm). Incorporation of radiolabel into DNA during synthesis or contamination of DNA with other radiolabelled macromolecules cannot be excluded.

It was not possible to trap any alkylating metabolites *in vitro* with 4-(4-nitrobenzyl)-pyridine, following incubation of vinylidene chloride with a mouse liver microsomal system [15].

8.5.2 Genotoxicity in bacteria

The mutagenicity of vinylidene chloride in bacteria has been demonstrated by a number of research workers and has been related to the asymmetry of the putative epoxide metabolite [73]. The positive effect was not seen in every study (Table 9) and in some cases this may have been due to volatilization of the compound. Vinylidene chloride (of unspecified purity) in air at 0.2, 2, or 20% for 4 h induced revertants (gene mutations) in the TA1530 and TA100 strains of *Salmonella typhimurium* in the presence of NADPH-supplemented 9000-g liver supernatant (S9) from phenobarbital pretreated male OF-1 mice. Mutagenicity towards TA100 was also catalysed by mouse kidney and lung 9000-g supernatants [14]. These authors demonstrated that mutagenicity was not due to the stabilizer 4-methoxyphenol. The role of cytochrome P-450 in metabolic activation was evident from the lack of mutagenicity in the absence of NADPH and from the observed greater mutagenicity of vinylidene chloride towards *S. typhimurium* TA100 when mice used for S9 donation were pretreated with phenobarbital. The role of reactive electrophiles in mutagenicity was supported by the marked inhibition of mutagenicity by the nucleophiles *N*-acetyl-cysteine and *N*-acetyl-methionine. Protection against bacterial mutagenesis was also afforded by pretreatment of rats (which provided the hepatic S9) with pregnenolone-16 α-carnonitrile, amino-cetonitrile, or disulfiram [15]. The mechanism(s) of these effects are not known but may be via increased detoxification of vinylidene chloride or its metabolites. In this study, 3-methylcholanthrene as well as phenobarbital pretreatment of rats provided S9 that had up to 2-fold greater capacity than untreated rat liver preparations to activate vinylidene chloride (99% pure) to bacterial mutagens. Liver specimens showing no pathological lesions, obtained from 4 adult human patients for diagnostic purposes provided S9 fractions that activated vinylidene chloride to mutagens detected by *S. typhimurium* TA100 at approximately one-fifth the activity of untreated mouse liver S9.

Jones & Hathaway [101] found vinylidene chloride (unspecified purity) to be only very weakly mutagenic in *S. typhimurium* strain TA1535 in the presence of liver (1.6 × background) and kidney (2.3 × background) S9 from untreated male Alderley Park Swiss-derived albino mice. Exposure was via the atmosphere (5% vinylidene chloride for 72 h) inside gas-tight culture vessels. Use of S9 from mice pretreated with Aroclor 1254 enhanced mutagenicity in the test. In contrast, liver S9 preparations from male Sprague-Dawley rats were able to mediate mutagenicity only after Aroclor pretreatment and at a mutation frequency approximately 25% of that seen with the corresponding mouse S9. These data are in agreement with the greater oxidative metabolism observed in the mouse compared with the rat (section 6.1.4). In this study, liver S9 from uninduced marmoset or from a single, apparently uninduced, human subject was not able to mediate the bacterial mutagenicity of vinylidene chloride, though a positive result was obtained using a liver S9 from a human subject who had received long-term phenobarbital medication. Thus, human beings appear to be more similar to rats than to mice with respect to hepatic metabolic activation of vinylidene chloride.

Exposure of *S. typhimurium* strain TA100 to 2% vinylidene chloride (99% pure) in air in the presence of a hepatic S9 fraction from untreated or phenobarbital-pretreated male OF-1 mice caused a linear increase in the mutagenic response up to 4 h of exposure [137]. This was in agreement with the dependence of bacterial mutagenicity on duration of exposure shown by Waskell [239]. Again, phenobarbital pretreatment enhanced the metabolic activation.

Oesch et al. [156] detected the mutagenicity of vinylidene chloride (99.996% pure) with *S. typhimurium* strains TA1535, TA1537, TA92, TA100, TA98, and *Escherichia coli* strain WP2 *uvrA* following exposure to vinylidene chloride in the atmosphere for 4 h at 1500–90 000 mg/m^3 (375–22 500 ppm) and with an NADPH-fortified liver S9 fraction from untreated male Swiss-Webster mice as an activation system. Again, it was established that the inhibitor, methoxyphenol, was not mutagenic. A comparative study was made of kidney and liver S9 fractions from different species regarding their ability to activate vinylidene chloride to mutagens detected by *S. typhimurium* strain TA100. The order of ability to mediate mutagenesis was as follows: male and female Swiss-Webster and C57BL/6J Han mouse liver and Chinese hamster (Fue:FUST) liver > Sprague-Dawley rat liver > human liver > Chinese hamster kidney > male mouse kidney (both strains) > rat kidney and female mouse kidney. Metabolic activation was not accomplished or was very weak in the last two tissue samples. As with the study by Bartsch et al. [14], mutagenicity was inhibited by a nucleophile (in this case glutathione) and it was also found not to be affected by the addition of purified microsomal epoxide hydrolase to the test. Despite changes in drug-metabolizing enzymes as a result of pretreatment of rats and mice with vinylidene chloride (section 8.2.1), S9 fractions derived from treated animals were not found to have a greater metabolic activation capacity in the mutagenicity assay.

The mutagenicity of vinylidene chloride towards *S. typhimurium* TA100 was detected by Baden et al. [10, 11, 12] not only following gaseous exposure for 8 h at a level of 3% but also after incubation in suspension at 3% for up to 2 h. In agreement with the data given above, Aroclor pretreatment of rats enhanced the ability of liver S9 to mediate vinylidene chloride mutagenicity and human liver S9 was also capable of catalysing the formation of mutagens. The mutagenicity of vinylidene chloride (unspecified purity) in liquid suspension assays (2.5 mmol vinylidene chloride/litre; 2 h incubation) was also shown to be positive by Greim et al. [64], as evidenced by reverse gene mutation at one locus in *E. coli* strain K12. When monitored for reverse gene mutation at 2 other loci, or forward mutation at 1 locus, a negative result was obtained, but only one dose level was used in this study.

Results of spot tests with *S. typhimurium* strains TA1950, TA1951, TA1952, TA1535, TA1538, TA100, and TA98 were reported briefly by Cerna & Kypenova [26]. Vinylidene chloride (unspecified purity) was added to plates at 1, 10, and 100% in DMSO (0.05 ml). At 100%, vinylidene chloride produced reversion of both base substitution and frame-shift mutations in the absence of a metabolic activation system. When tested in a host-mediated assay (female ICR mice) at doses quoted as LD_{50} and 50% LD_{50}, a significant increase in the revertants of *S. typhimurium* TA1950, TA1951, and TA1952 was reported that was inversely related to dose.

A further brief report was given by McCarroll et al. [129] in which vinylidene chloride (1.6 and 3%, "metabolically activated doses") was shown to be markedly mutagenic to *S. typhimurium* TA1535 and TA100 in a microfluctuation assay involving a 72-h exposure.

Chloroacetic acid, a metabolite of vinylidene chloride, was found not to be mutagenic to *S. typhimurium* strains TA100, TA1535, TA1537, TA1538, and TA98 using a plate incorporation protocol without the addition of an S9 system [128]. Chloroacetic acid did not cause mutagenicity in *S. typhimurium* strain TA1530 in the presence or absence of S9 from phenobarbital-pretreated mice [136].

8.5.3 Genotoxicity in yeast

Bronzetti et al. [19] studied the mutagenicity of vinylidene chloride (99.57% pure) in yeast. Vinylidene chloride (0-50 mmol/litre for 2 h preincubation in suspension) did not induce reverse gene point mutation or produce mitotic gene conversion in a diploid strain (D7) of *Saccharomyces cerevisiae* in the absence of a microsomal activation system. However, in the presence of a post-mitochondrial supernatant from mice pretreated with Aroclor 1254, a dose-related induction of revertants and convertants was seen between 30 and 50 mmol vinylidene chloride/litre. Genotoxicity was also examined in yeast exposed to vinylidene chloride in an intrasanguinous host-mediated assay. The host species i.e., male Swiss albino CD mice, were given vinylidene chloride orally in an acute single dose study (400 mg/kg) or in a short-term study (100 mg/kg, 5 days per week followed by 200 mg/kg on the day of the assay). The yeast cells (4 x 10^8) were injected via the retro-orbital sinus immediately before the administration of vinylidene chloride on the day of the assay and were recovered from various organs 4 h later. A positive result for the induction of revertants and convertants was found for yeast cells recovered from the liver and kidneys, but the results were negative or only very weakly positive for both parameters in cells from the lung.

8.5.4 Genotoxicity in plants

After exposure to 5152 mg vinylidene chloride/m^3 (1288 ppm) for 6 h, inactivation of a dominant gene (forward mutation) in *Tradescantia* (hybrid clone 4430) was not observed [228]. However, at 88 mg vinylidene chloride/m^3 (22 ppm) for 24 h, a positive result was recorded. Although this finding indicates the potential for mutagenicity in plants, the dose-response relationship needs to be clarified.

8.5.5 Genotoxicity in mammalian cells in vitro

Costa & Ivanetich [33] investigated the effects of vinylidene chloride (unspecified purity) on DNA repair (unscheduled DNA synthesis) in isolated hepatocytes from male Long-Evans rats that had been pretreated with phenobarbital. When administered to hepatocytes at a maximum subtoxic dose level (2.1 mmol/litre), vinylidene chloride stimulated unscheduled DNA synthesis as shown by enhanced incorporation of deoxy-[5-^{3}H]-cytidine into DNA.

However, the mutagenicity of vinylidene chloride was found to be negative when tested at two loci (induction of resistance to 8-azaguanine and ouabain) in V79 Chinese hamster cells in the presence of a post-mitochondrial supernatant from phenobarbital pretreated rats and mice [43]. In this test, the V79 cells were exposed to 2 and 10% vinylidene chloride (unspecified purity) in air for 5 h. This treatment led to dose-dependent cytotoxicity in the presence of rat but not mouse liver post-mitochondrial fractions. Using a similar protocol, Huberman et al. [82] demonstrated that the vinylidene chloride metabolite, monochloroacetic acid, in accordance with negative mutagenicity in bacteria (section 8.5.2), did not show any activity in inducing 8-azaguanine and ouabain resistant mutants in Chinese hamster V79 cells, when tested up to a level of 2.5 mmol/litre.

In a survey of the cytogenetic effects of 60 chemicals on cultured mammalian cells, Sasaki et al. [193] reported that vinylidene chloride (3×10^{-2} and 3×10^{-3} mol/litre) failed to produce chromosomal breaks in Chinese hamster (Don 6) cells. A microsomal metabolic system was not included in the assay. Other research workers have also carried out cytogenetic studies on mammalian cells *in vitro*. McCarroll et al. [129] analysed Chinese hamster ovary cells (CHO) for sister chromatid exchange following exposure to vinylidene chloride (unspecified purity). Consistent and dose-related increases resulted from a 24-h exposure to atmospheres containing 1.8, 3.6, 5.4, or 7% vinylidene chloride. Only at 7% was the effect significant and shorter exposure periods provided negative results. In this brief report it was not stated whether a mammalian hepatic microsomal fraction was included in the study. Sawada et al. [196] also investigated the ability of vinylidene chloride (99% pure) to induce chromosomal aberrations and sister chromatid exchange in a Chinese hamster cell line (CHL). Cells were treated for 6 h with a range of dose levels between 0 and 2 mg/ml, at which toxicity was observed. In the presence of a liver S9 fraction from PCB (KC-400)-pretreated male F344 rats, vinylidene chloride gave a relatively weak, but significant, increase in the incidence of sister chromatid exchanges. The result was negative in the absence of S9. The findings were similar when chromosomal aberrations were used as an end point for genetic toxicity. In the presence (but not in the absence) of S9, a dose-dependent induction of chromosomal aberrations was seen (14% aberrant cells at 0.25 mg/ml and 54% at 1.5 mg/ml). These effects were not elicited by p-methoxyphenol (the inhibitor). The role of cytochrome P-450 in the metabolic activation of vinylidene chloride was shown by the inhibition of the enhancement of aberrations with metyrapone and a protective effect was seen by the addition of glutathione. Two metabolites of vinylidene chloride, chloroacetyl chloride and chloroacetic acid, were negative in these tests in support of the theory that vinylidene chloride oxide may be the active genotoxic metabolite.

8.5.6 Genotoxicity in mammalian cells *in vivo*

Evidence for the detectable but minimal covalent binding of [^{14}C]-vinylidene chloride *in vivo* has already been discussed [186] (sections 8.1.1.2 and 8.5.1). As part of this study, the ability of vinylidene chloride to induce unscheduled DNA synthesis (DNA repair) was also investigated in mice. The measurement of DNA repair by the uptake of [^{3}H]-thymidine into DNA was hampered by incomplete inhibition of replicative DNA synthesis by hydroxyurea.

Though unscheduled DNA synthesis was minimal, the slight increase was statistically significant in mouse kidney at the 200 mg vinylidene chloride/m^3 (50 ppm) exposure level.

Short et al. [203] investigated the incidence of germinal mutations of the dominant lethal type in 11 male CD rats exposed through inhalation of 220 mg vinylidene chloride/m^3 (55 ppm) for 6 h/day and 5 days/week. During week 11 of exposure, the treated animals were housed with 2 virgin females until mating had taken place. Neither pre-implantation nor post-implantation losses were observed in the pregnancies that resulted from mating with vinylidene chloride-exposed males; thus, dominant lethal mutations were not produced. Anderson et al. [3] also did not find any evidence for a dominant lethal effect. Male CD-1 mice were exposed by inhalation to 40, 120, or 200 mg vinylidene chloride/m^3 (10, 30, and 50 ppm), for 6 h/day, over 5 days. Fifteen or 16 days after caging the males with untreated females (over a 2-month period), the females were killed for examination of the uteri. As a result of toxicity, only 6/20 and 18/20 male mice survived exposure to vinylidene chloride at 200 and 120 mg/m^3 (50 and 30 ppm), respectively. No effects were seen in the frequency of pregnancy or in the number of post-implantational early fetal deaths. There was also no evidence of pre-implantational egg losses as indicated by the total implants/pregnant female.

A number of *in vivo* cytogenetic studies reported on vinylidene chloride have been unable to show a significant positive response. In the inhalation study by Lee et al. [118] (details given in sections 8.3.1 and 8.7.1), cytogenetic analysis of bone marrow revealed no change following exposure of CD-1 mice or CD rats to 220 mg vinylidene chloride/m^3 (55 ppm), for 6 h/day, 5 days/week, for up to 12 months. Cerna & Kypenova [26] gave single and repeated (1 dose per day for 5 days) ip doses of vinylidene chloride to female ICR mice. Neither a single dose (quoted as 1/2 LD$_{50}$) nor repeated doses (quoted as 1/6 LD$_{50}$) induced chromosomal aberrations. In the long-term study by Quast et al. [178] (section 8.3.1 for details), cytogenetic evaluations on 4 rats/sex exposed to 0, 100, or 300 mg vinylidene chloride/m^3 (0, 25, or 75 ppm) for 6 months did not show any adverse effects. A negative *in vivo* cytogenetic effect was also borne out by the work of Sawada et al. [196]. In this study, 6 male ddY mice per group were given vinylidene chloride (99% pure) by gavage, either as a single dose (0–200 mg/kg) or as 4 doses (1–100 mg/kg each) given at 24-h intervals. No increase in the frequency of micronucleated erythrocytes was observed in the bone marrow. A micronucleus test in the liver and blood of fetuses in vinylidene chloride-treated mice was also negative (section 8.6). These authors suggest that, in contrast to the *in vitro* studies where positive genotoxicity has been found, the life time of the reactive metabolites of vinylidene chloride may be too short for a sufficient amount to have reached the target cells analysed *in vivo*.

However, this conclusion conflicts with the findings of Hofmann & Peh [77] who studied chromosome aberrations in 50 metaphase bone marrow cells of 4 male and 5 female Chinese hamsters after short-term inhalation (6 h/day, 5 days/week for 6 weeks) of either 120 or 400 mg vinylidene chloride/m^3 (30 or 100 ppm). In comparison with control groups (fresh air), there was no effect on mortality but 7–8 times more aberrations were observed in the animals exposed to 120 mg vinylidene chloride/m^3 (30 ppm) and 9–10 times more aberrations were seen at the 400 mg/m^3 (100 ppm) dose level. Using the same technique for analysis of chromosomal aberrations, Zeller & Peh [247] studied the effects of a single oral dose (216 mg/kg) in Chinese hamsters. Animals that were killed 6 h after dosing showed a higher number of aberrations (1.6%) than animals given the same doses and killed after 24 h (1.2%) and 48 h (1.4%). The untreated control animals showed the lowest rate of aberrations (0.6%). No statistical test was carried out.

8.5.7 Summary

Data on mutagenicity and other short-term tests for carcinogenicity are summarized in Table 9. Genotoxicity has been observed in prokaryotic (in the presence of mammalian enzymes) and eukaryotic cells *in vitro*. However, genotoxicity was not observed in the majority of tests carried out on mammals *in vivo*. Reports of an effect in the latter are restricted to the observation of chromosomal aberrations in the bone marrow cells of Chinese hamsters and the finding of a slight increase in DNA repair in the mouse kidney.

Table 9. Summary of genotoxicity data for vinylidene chloride

Test system/End point of analysis	Metabolizing system	Dose range	Result[a]	Reference
PROKARYOTES IN VITRO *Salmonella typhimurium* (reverse gene mutation)				
Strains TA 100, TA 1530	+ phenobarbital-induced mouse kidney, liver, and lung S9 mix	0.2–20% in air for 4 h	+ ve	[14, 15]
Strain TA 100	+ phenobarbital-induced mouse liver S9 (-NADPH)	0.2–20% in air for 4 h	- ve	[14, 15]
Strain TA 100	+ human liver S9 mix	2% in air for 4 h	+ ve	[15]
Strain TA 1530	+ phenobarbital or 3-methyl cholanthrene-induced rat liver S9	2% or 20% in air for 4 h	+ ve	[15]
Strains TA 100, TA 1535, TA 98, TA 1537 "blind study", preincubation	± rat or hamster S9 mix (Aroclor induced)	0–3333 µg/plate	- ve	[146]
Strain TA 100	± Aroclor-induced rat liver S9 mix	3% for 2 or 8 h	+ ve	[10, 11, 12]
Strains TA 1950, TA 1951, TA 1952, TA 1535, TA 1538 TA 100, TA 98 (spot test)	None	1, 10, and 100% in DMSO (0.05 ml/plate)	+ ve at 100% dose	[26]
Strains TA 1535, TA 1537, TA 92, TA 100, TA 98	+ mouse liver S9 mix	1500–90 000 mg/m^3 for 4 h	+ ve	[156]

Table 9 (contd).

Strain TA 100	+ liver and kidney S9 mix from mouse, rat, Chinese hamster. Also human liver S9 mix	360-50 000 mg/m³ for 4 h	+ ve (except where S9 obtained from female mouse kidney and rat kidney)	[156]
Strain TA 1535	+ mouse liver and kidney S9 mix	5% for 72 h	+ ve (induction of S9 increased response)	[103]
	+ uninduced rat liver S9 mix or marmoset or human S9 mix	5% for 72 h	- ve	[103]
	+ induced rat liver S9 mix	5% for 72 h	+ ve	[103]
	+ uninduced marmoset liver S9 mix	5% for 72 h	- ve	[103]
	+ uninduced human liver S9 mix	5% for 72 h	- ve	[103]
	+ phenobarbital-induced human liver S9 mix	5% for 72 h	+ ve	[103]

Table 9 (contd).

Test system/End point of analysis	Metabolizing system	Dose range	Result[a]	Reference
Escherichia coli (Reverse gene mutation)				
Strain WP2 uvr A	+ mouse liver S9 mix	1500–90 000 mg/m^3 for 4 h	+ ve	[156]
Strain K12 (Forward and reverse gene liquid suspension mutation)	–	2.5 mmol/litre	+ ve (for 1 locus only)	[64]
PROKARYOTES IN VIVO *Salmonella typhimurium* Strains TA 1950, TA 1951 TA 1952 host mediated in ICR mice	–	at LD$_{50}$ and half-LD$_{50}$ dose	+ ve	[26]
EUKARYOTES IN VITRO *Saccharomyces* (yeast) (reverse gene mutation and gene conversion)	± Aroclor-induced rat liver S9 mix	0–50 mmol/litre for 2 h preincubation	+ ve (– ve without S9)	[19]
Chinese hamster V79 cells (forward gene mutation)	± Aroclor-induced rat liver S9 mix	2, 20% for 2 h	– ve	[43]
Chinese hamster V79 cells (chromosomal breaks)		3×10^{-2} or 3×10^{-3} mmol/litre	– ve	[193]

Table 9 (contd).

System	S9	Dose	Result	Ref
Chinese hamster ovary cells (sister chromatid exchange)		1.8-7% atmosphere for 24 h	+ ve	[129]
Chinese hamster ovary cells (sister chromatid exchange)	± Aroclor-induced rat liver S9 mix	0-2 mg/ml	+ ve (weak response)	[196]
Primary hepatocytes from phenobarbital-treated rats (unscheduled DNA synthesis)		2.1 mmol/litre (maximum subtoxic dose)	+ ve	[32]
EUKARYOTES *IN VIVO*				
Tradescantia (flower) (forward gene mutation)		88 and 5152 mg/m^3	+ ve (at lower dose only)	[228]
Saccharomyces (host mediated assay in Swiss mice)		400 mg/kg or 5x100 mg/kg daily plus 200 mg/kg on last day	+ ve for yeast cells recovered from liver and kidneys, but not from lung	[19]
CD-1 mice and Sprague-Dawley rats (DNA adduct formation in liver and kidney)		rats: 40 mg/m^3 mice: 40 or 200 mg/m^3 for 6 h	+ ve (but minimal binding detected) mouse > rat kidney > liver	[186]

Table 9 (contd).

Test system/End point of analysis	Metabolizing system	Dose range	Result[a]	Reference
CD-1 mice (unscheduled DNA synthesis in liver and kidney)	-	200 mg/m³ for 6 h	+ve (but minimal); effect observed in kidneys only	[186]
CD-1 mice (bone marrow cytogenetics)	-	220 mg/m³ for 6 h, 5 days/week for 12 months	-ve	[118]
CD rats (bone marrow cytogenetics)	-	220 mg/m³ for 6 h, 5 days/week for 12 months	-ve	[118]
Rats (male and female) (bone marrow cytogenetics)		0, 100, or 300 mg/m³ for 6 months	-ve	[178]
ICR mice (bone marrow cytogenetics)	-	One-half LD_{50} one-sixth LD_{50} × 5 days	-ve	[26]
Male ddY mice (bone marrow micronucleus assay)	-	0–200 mg/kg or 0–100 mg/kg × 4 by gavage	-ve	[196]

Table 9 (contd).

Chinese hamster (bone marrow cytogenetics)		120 or 400 mg/m^3 (30 or 100 ppm) 6 h/day, 5 days/week for 6 weeks	+ ve [77]
CD-1 mice (male) (dominant lethal assay)	-	40, 120, 200 mg/m^3 6 h/day for 5 days	- ve [3]
CD rats (dominant lethal assay)	-	220 mg/m^3, 6 h/day 5 days/week for 11 weeks	- ve [203]

[a] + ve = positive response.
    - ve = negative response.

8.6 Reproduction, Embryotoxicity, and Teratogenicity

Details of studies on dominant lethality in rats and mice are given in section 8.5.6. These results provide no evidence for an adverse effect on male reproduction. The fertility of male and female Sprague-Dawley rats and neonatal toxicity were investigated in a 3-generation, 2-litter study [151] in which test animals were continuously given drinking-water containing 0, 50, 100, or 200 mg vinylidene chloride/litre (99.5% minimum purity). Ten male and 20 female F_0 rats were treated and 15 male and 30 female rats were used in the control F_0 groups. These animals were mated after 100 days exposure (to provide F_{1a} litters) and again 10 days after weaning of the first litter (to provide F_{1b} litters). Parents for the F_2 and F_3 generations were selected randomly from the F_{1b} and F_2 litters, respectively. They were mated at 110 days of age to produce the F_2 and F_{3a} litters, respectively. The F_2 rats were then remated 10 days after weaning of the F_{3a} and F_{3b} litters to produce the F_{3b} and F_{3c} litters, respectively. No evidence was found for an effect of vinylidene chloride on fertility, though marked fluctuations in the fertility index in all groups including the controls made interpretation of the results difficult. Neonatal survival was lower in the F_2 and F_{3a} litters of dams ingesting vinylidene chloride than in the respective control groups but not lower than that of the historical data for the laboratory. Furthermore, reduced survival in some litters was followed by normal survival in subsequent litters from the same adults. It was concluded that the decreased survival was due to chance. Necropsies were carried out on rats found dead or moribund, all weanlings not selected for future matings, and F_1 and F_2 adults after the litters were weaned.

Absolute and relative kidney weights of weanling rats were comparable with controls. No organ weight changes related to treatment were seen in F_1 adults but elevated relative liver weights of female rats ingesting 200 mg vinylidene chloride/litre were seen in the F_2 generation. An increase in serum glutamic pyruvic transaminase (25% above control mean) was observed in female F_2 rats at the 200 mg/litre level.

Signs of mild hepatotoxicity (fatty liver) were seen at treatment levels of 100 mg vinylidene chloride/litre and 200 mg/litre in F_1 and F_2 rats and the incidence of chronic renal disease (though high in controls) was greater in male rats treated with 200 mg vinylidene chloride/litre than in control animals. Nitschke et al. [151] concluded that vinylidene chloride treatment did not significantly affect the reproductive capacity of rats.

Sawada et al. [196] investigated the incidence of micronuclei in fetal liver and fetal erythrocytes 24 h following exposure of pregnant ICR mice to 0, 25, 50, or 100 mg vinylidene chloride/kg (given by intraperitoneal injection). No significant increase in micronuclei in these cells was observed as a result of treatment, and the results did not show any evidence of a transplacental passage of genotoxic metabolites or precursors.

In a study on Charles River CD rats (18–20 per dose group) and CD-1 mice (7–24 per dose group), Short et al. [202] exposed animals to vinylidene chloride through inhalation at 60–1796 mg/m^3 (15–449 ppm), for 22–23 h/day during various periods of organogenesis. On day 20 (rats) or day 17 (mice) of gestation, fetal abnormalities were seen at all dose levels in rats and a high incidence of early and complete resorptions was seen in mice exposed to vinylidene chloride concentrations ≥ 120 mg/m^3 (30 ppm). However, these effects were associated with a decreased weight gain and increased mortality in the dams. Since similar fetal abnormalities of the soft tissues and skeleton occurred in a feed-restricted group of mice, the defects may be attributed to maternal toxicity. In rats, malformations were seen in all groups and hydrocephalus was significantly increased in a dose-related manner from 2.5% in controls, 7.3% at 60 mg/m^3 (15 ppm), 15.1% at 228 mg/m^3 (57 ppm) to 33.3% at 1200 mg/m^3 (300 ppm). Retarded ossification was seen in all treated groups. Early resorptions were significantly increased from 2% in controls to 49% at 228 mg/m^3 (57 ppm) and 64% at 1796 mg/m^3 (449 ppm). Fetal weight was reduced in a dose-related manner and the reductions were significant at 228, 1200, and 1796 mg/m^3 (57, 300, and 449 ppm). Food-restricted controls showed reduced fetal weight and retarded ossification but no significant increase in resorption rate or in the frequency of hydrocephalus. Aspects of maternal toxicity may be responsible for these effects. Part of this study involved an investigation of behavioural changes in Charles River CD rats (19 or 20 per dose group). The rats were exposed to 224 or 1132 mg vinylidene chloride/m^3 (56 or 283 ppm) for 22–23 h/day, on days 8–20 of gestation. A dose-related weight loss over this period indicated maternal toxicity and the body weight of pups from the rats treated with 1132 mg/m^3 (283 ppm) were lower than control weights (as with pups from feed-restricted rats). Two groups of 3 pups/dose level and per sex were observed for activity in a maze for 2–4 months after birth. Also one animal of each sex per dose level from each litter was subjected to pre-weaning behavioural and physical maturation tests. Maze activity was not affected by the vinylidene chloride treatment, nor were startle response, bar holding or swimming ability. However, surface righting ability was delayed in pups from treated rats. Tooth production was delayed in pups from the rats treated with 1132 mg/m^3 (283 ppm) (as in feed-restricted rats) but opening of the external ear was more rapid than in control pups. In conclusion, the only adverse effects bserved could be attributed to maternal toxicity. Murray et al. [1979] investigated embryonic and fetal development in rats and rabbits following inhalation or oral ingestion (rats only) of vinylidene chloride (minimum purity 99.5%) during gestation. In the inhalation studies, Sprague-Dawley rats (30–44 per dose group) and New Zealand White rabbits (18–20 per dose group) were exposed to 640, 320, or 80 (rats only) mg vinylidene chloride/m^3 (160, 80, or 20 ppm), for 7 h/day, from days 6 to 15 (rats) and days 6 to18 (rabbits) of gestation. Groups of 20–47 pregnant rats and 16 pregnant rabbits served as controls for each dose level. For the ingestion study, 26 pregnant rats (24 controls) received drinking-water containing vinylidene chloride at 200 mg/litre (approximately 40 mg/kg per day) from days 6 to 15 of gestation. Cesarean section was carried out on day 21 and day 29 for rats and rabbits, respectively.

Although a teratogenic effect was not observed, some evidence of embryotoxicity and fetotoxicity was seen in rats and rabbits. In the rat inhalation study, there was delayed ossification and a dose-related increased incidence of wavy ribs at 320 and 640 mg/m^3 (80 and 160 ppm), concentrations that were toxic to the dams. At 80 mg/m^3 (20 ppm), a concentration that was not maternally toxic, no embryo- or fetotoxic effects were seen. In the rabbits, a dose of 640 mg/m^3 (160 ppm) produced weight loss in the dams, increased resorptions, increased incidence of 13 pairs of ribs and delayed ossification of the fifth sternebra. At 320 mg/m^3 (80 ppm), there was no effect on dams or fetuses.

8.7 Carcinogenicity

Details of a number of the studies described here have been provided in section 8.4. In such cases, only an outline of the experimental protocol is given.

8.7.1 Inhalation

In a long-term inhalation study (220 mg vinylidene chloride/m^3 (55 ppm)) carried out by Lee et al. [118, 119] (section 8.3.1 for details of treatments), haemangiosarcomas in the mesenteric lymph node or subcutaneous tissue were reported in 2 treated male rats and hepatic haemangiosarcomas were found in 2 male and 1 female mice in the treatment group. No haemangiosarcomas were seen in control animals. Small bronchioalveolar adenomas were also reported in 6 male mice (17%) compared with 1 in the control group of male mice (4%). The significance of this finding was considered questionable since, according to other reports, such adenomas, which occurred relatively late in the study, were common in untreated mice. The numbers of animals used in the treatment and control groups in this study were very low (16 or less per group after 9 months) and the study was limited to 12 months, which is inadequate. Furthermore, the authors referred to the spontaneous occurrence of hepatomas in mice at a similar age in other reports. In a follow-up study, it was not possible to repeat the finding of an increase in tumour incidence [79]. Intermittent exposure was limited to up to 10 months (rats) and up to 6 months (mice) at a vinylidene chloride concentration of 220 mg/m^3 (55 ppm) (details given in section 8.3.1), and was followed by a 12-month observation period. In contrast to the results of Lee et al. [119], no tumours arose in the treated animals other than spontaneous tumours expected on the basis of their incidence in control animals. In this study also, a small number of animals were used (14–16 rats and 12 mice per sex for 10-and 6-month treatments, respectively) and exposures were limited to periods of less than 12 months for both species.

The results of a number of other long-term inhalation studies on rats suggest a lack of carcinogenicity of vinylidene chloride in this species, but, as explained, these reports are not conclusive. Viola & Caputo [229] investigated the incidence of tumours in 51 male and 23 female Wistar rats exposed to 800 mg vinylidene chloride/m^3 (200 ppm) for 4 h/day, 5 days/week, for 5 months. For the following 7 months, the concentration was reduced to 400 mg/m^3 (100 ppm) because of toxicity. The animals were then given a complete autopsy at spontaneous death or after being killed when moribund. Sprague-Dawley rats were also examined after exposure to 400 mg/m^3 (100 ppm) (30 of each sex) and 300 mg/m^3 (75 ppm) (16 and 21 male and female rats, respectively). Thirty control rats of each sex were used for each strain. "No grossly observable correlation between tumour formation and vinylidene chloride inhalation" was seen but a final report following the completion of microscopic examination of tissues and organs has not been released. A more substantial study has been reported in several stages [134, 178, 179, 180]. The details of the long-term inhalation study on rats are given in section 8.3.1. In outline, following the first month of treatment, animals of a relatively large group (minimum of 84 rats/sex per dose group) were treated intermittently with levels of up to 300 mg vinylidene chloride/m^3 (75 ppm) for the substantial period of 18 months and were sacrificed at 24 months. The total incidence of tumours was similar in control and dosed animals, though the incidences of several tumours and/or tumour types were found to be statistically increased compared with the controls ($P \leq 0.05$, Fisher's Exact Probability Test). These were not attributed to vinylidene chloride exposure on the basis of comparable historical control data.

The carcinogenicity of vinylidene chloride by inhalation was studied by Maltoni et al. [139, 141] in rats, mice, and hamsters. The experimental details for the long-term study are given in section 8.3.1. The intermittent exposure levels were up to 100 mg/m^3 (up to 25 ppm) (hamsters), 600 reduced from 800 mg/m^3, (150 reduced from 200 ppm) (rats), and 100 mg/m^3 (25 ppm) (mice) and were given over a period of 52 weeks. The dose levels in rats and mice were limited by toxicity (section 8.3.1). Animals were then observed until spontaneous death. Tumour incidence in hamsters was not increased by treatment with vinylidene chloride. The only type of tumour in treated rats for which the incidence was greater than that in the controls was in the mammary gland, but a dose-response relationship was not observed and the authors suspected "non-specific factors" (linked to inhalation) to be responsible. As part of the same project, Maltoni et al. [140] specifically investigated the ability of vinylidene chloride to produce brain tumours in Sprague-Dawley rats. Groups of 30 rats of each sex were exposed to 40, 100, 200, or 400 mg vinylidene chloride/m^3 (10, 25, 50, or 100 ppm), and 60 rats per sex to 600 mg/m^3 (150 ppm), for 4 h/day, 4–5 days weekly, for 52 weeks (100 control rats were used per sex). No evidence for the induction of brain tumours (ependymomas, gliomas, or meningiomas) was found.

A number of tumour-types were observed in mice [139, 141] including kidney adenocarcinomas, mammary tumours, pulmonary adenomas, and leukaemias. The incidence of both mammary and pulmonary tumours (mainly adenomas) was statistically higher in treated mice compared with the controls (tested by the rank test of Krauth, Fisher's Exact Probability Test, Logrank test and probit analysis [142]. As with rats, non-specific factors may have been responsible. However, a dose-response relationship was not observed in either case. Kidney adenocarcinoma (a rare tumour in mice) was observed in 29 (28 male) out of 257 mice (300 at start) treated with 100 mg vinylidene chloride/m^3 (25 ppm) and in 2 out of the 18 male surviving mice treated with 200 mg/m^3 (50 ppm). Kidney adenocarcinomas were not seen in the 14 surviving females at 200 mg/m^3 (50 ppm), in mice treated with 40 mg/m^3 (10 ppm) (0/60), or in control mice (0/380).

Maltoni et al. [142] exposed two groups of approximately 60 male and 60 female Sprague-Dawley rats to vinylidene chloride transplacentally, continuing the exposure by inhalation at birth (see Table 10, pp. 114–120). Treatment of dams with vinylidene chloride at 400 mg/m^3 (100 ppm) through inhalation for 4 h/day, 5 days/week, was started when embryos were 12 days of age. The inhalation treatment of dams and offspring was continued after birth with exposure to 400 mg vinylidene chloride/m^3 (100 ppm) for 7 h/day, 5 days/week over 8 or 97 weeks, giving a total exposure period of 15 or 104 weeks. Offspring may also have been exposed via ingestion of milk at the suckling stage.

An increased incidence of malignant neoplasias of the haemolymphoreticular system, generally classified as leukaemia, was observed in both males and females of both groups exposed to vinylidene chloride. A slight decrease in body weight was also reported in these animals. Although a quadrupling of leukaemia incidence appeared to occur in female rats and a doubling of these tumours occurred in the male rats, very little other information was reported. It is possible that a few of the tumours called "leukaemia" are histiocytic sarcomas and should be classified separately from leukaemias. Unless this is known, the contribution of this finding to the overall data base is compromised. The authors pointed out that a considerable increase in total malignant tumours occurred in the rats exposed to vinylidene chloride for 104 weeks, when the treatment was started prenatally. In contrast, a 52-week exposure of rats beginning in young adulthood (see above), showed no increased incidence of leukaemia at exposures as high as 600 mg/m^3 (150 ppm) for 52 weeks, and only a "borderline" increase in total malignant tumours. Both age at the start of exposure and the length of exposure appear to be important factors influencing tumour development in Sprague-Dawley rats exposed to vinylidene chloride.

Laib et al. [114] investigated the occurrence of putative preneoplastic nodules in the liver of rats treated with vinylidene chloride. Neonate Wistar rats were exposed, together with mothers, to vinylidene chloride in the air at 440 ± 60 mg/m^3 (110 ± 15 ppm) (8 h per day, 5 days per week). Exposure to this concentration, did not result in increased lethality or reduction in body and liver weights. Histochemical analysis of frozen liver sections, produced immediately after 6 weeks exposure, revealed ATPase-free islets, postulated to indicate preneoplasia.

8.7.2 Oral

There have been three studies on the oral carcinogenicity of vinylidene chloride in which a reasonable number of rats were given a range of dose levels for an adequate length of time. In the first [177, 179], vinylidene chloride was included in the drinking-water at a level up to 200 mg/litre (200 ppm) over a 2-year period (details given in section 8.3.2). No exposure-related neoplasms were detected. Although the incidence of mammary gland fibroadenomas/adenofibromas was greater in rats exposed to 50 mg/litre than in the control animals, this increase was not dose dependent and was within the range of the historical control data for untreated rats.

In the second study [139, 141], vinylidene chloride was given by gavage in olive oil (details of animals and dosing regimen are given in section 8.3.2). The intermittent dosing was over a period of 52 weeks and the animals were examined at spontaneous death. No increase in tumours was observed in treated rats and, in particular, there was no increased incidence of mammary tumours (these being considered due to "non-specific factors" when found in the corresponding inhalation study (section 8.7.1)).

In a third gavage study [154], doses of 1 and 5 mg/kg were given daily to rats for 2 years (details in section 8.3.2). No vinylidene chloride-related tumours were reported. In mice (section 8.3.2), given 2 or 10 mg/kg daily for 2 years, though the incidence of lymphomas was increased at the lower dose level ($P > 0.05$), this was not found at 10 mg/kg and thus does not appear to be related to vinylidene chloride exposure. However, the sponsors have recently found defects in the conduct of the study and it could not be satisfactorily evaluated.

A further study [172] was restricted to a single oral dose level given to BDIV rats throughout the life span from the time of weaning. The study also included oral dosing of the mothers during pregnancy. Twenty-four female pregnant rats were given vinylidene chloride orally (150 mg/kg) on the 17th day of gestation and their offspring (81 males and 64 females) were then treated weekly with 50 mg/kg (orally in olive oil) from the time of weaning. All survivors were killed at 120 weeks or when moribund and all major organs, as well as those that showed gross abnormalities, were examined histologically. Treatment did not increase the incidence of tumour-bearing animals, though liver tumours were increased in rats of both sexes (1/81 males and 3/80 females compared with 0/49 and 0/47 in male and female controls, respectively), and meningiomas were increased in males (6/81 compared with 1/49 in controls). The latter was found statistically to be not significant and, since a dose-response analysis was not possible, the results are inconclusive. In addition, hyperplastic nodules were found in the livers of 2/23 females given the single dose of vinylidene chloride during pregnancy and also in 2/81 males and 6/80 females among the progeny. There was a significant difference ($P = 0.04$) between treated and vehicle-treated control animals, no hyperplastic nodules being observed in the latter.

8.7.3 Other routes

Van Duuren et al. [227] studied the carcinogenicity of vinylidene chloride in groups of 30 female Ha: 1 CR Swiss mice following percutaneous and subcutaneous application compared with 100 untreated control animals. Following the application of vinylidene chloride at 121 mg/kg or 40 mg/kg in acetone to shaved dorsal skin, 3 times per week for between 440 and 594 days, animals were given a complete autopsy (except the cranial region) and abnormal-appearing tissues and organs were examined histologically. Routine sections of skin, liver, stomach, and kidney were also taken. Autopsies and additional sections from the injection site and liver were taken following the once weekly subcutaneous administration of 2 mg vinylidene chloride per mouse for the life span (78 weeks). Although in the percutaneous study, benign lung papillomas (19/30, 12/30 and 30/100) were seen at 121 mg/kg, 40 mg/kg, and 0 mg/kg, respectively, and stomach tumours were also observed at frequencies of 2/30, 0/30 and 5/100, respectively, the tumour incidence were not significantly elevated ($P > 0.05$; Chi-square analysis) in any of the treatment groups. However, when vinylidene chloride was given as an "initiating" agent (single dermal dose of 121 mg/kg) followed 14 days later with 5 µg of the "promoting" agent phorbol myristate acetate three times weekly, for 428–576 days, 8/30 mice developed papillomas compared with 9/120 and 6/90 in control (phorbol myristate acetate-treated) mice and 1/30 treated mice developed a squamous cell carcinoma compared with 1/120 and 2/90 in control mice treated with phorbol ester (2.5 and 5.0 µg, respectively). The incidence of papillomas in vinylidene chloride-treated mice was significantly greater than in the control groups ($P < 0.005$; Chi-square analysis). The authors concluded that "initiating" activity was shown with vinylidene chloride but that it was not a complete carcinogen. However, the finding of papillomas in the phorbol myristate acetate-treated control mice and the low number of animals used in the treatment groups make the interpretation of the results difficult.

8.7.4 Summary of carcinogenicity

A number of studies on rodents have been conducted that provide information on the potential carcinogenic action of vinylidene chloride (see Table 10). In these studies, vinylidene chloride was administered by inhalation, orally by gavage and in drinking-water, and by skin application and subcutaneous injection. Unfortunately, most of these studies were inadequate for the conclusive evaluation of carcinogenicity because of less than lifetime exposure regimens, insufficient numbers of animals, and an inadequate number of dose levels. Only some of the studies were designed and conducted as cancer biossays.

Increased tumour incidence was not found, in most of the studies, but there were the following exceptions. Kidney adenocarcinomas occurred in male Swiss mice exposed via inhalation to 100 or 200 mg vinylidene chloride/m^3 (25 or 50 ppm) but not to 40 mg/m^3 (10 ppm). This carcinogenic response may be related to the ability of vinylidene chloride to cause cytotoxic effects in the target organ (section 8.1.2 and 8.2.1). In addition to kidney adenocarcinomas, statistically significant excesses of mammary carcinomas were observed in female mice and pulmonary adenomas in mice of both sexes, but in these cases there was no dose-response relationship. In a 2-stage skin carcinogenicity assay in mice, there was some evidence that vinylidene chloride may have acted as an initiating agent.

In rats, an increase in mammary tumours that was not dose related was observed when adult animals were exposed through inhalation. In separate study groups, a slight increase in leukaemias was observed in rats exposed through inhalation *in utero* and then post-natally.

Table 10. Animal carcinogenicity studies[a]

Species/strain (Reference)	Route (Vehicle)	Number of animals in each group male / female	Dose	Duration of administration	Post-exposure period	Result male	female
Rat, Sprague-Dawley [139,141]	inhalation	100 / 100 30 / 30 30 / 30 30 / 30 60 / 60	0 mg/m^3 (0 ppm) 40 mg/m^3 (10 ppm) 100 mg/m^3 (25 ppm) 200 mg/m^3 (50 ppm) 600 mg/m^3 (150 ppm)	4 h/day, 4–5 days/week, 52 weeks	to spontaneous death	- - - - -	- - - - -
Rat, Sprague-Dawley [142] (in utero and post-natal exposure)	inhalation					*Leukemia*	*Leukemia*
		158 / 149[c]	0 mg/m^3 (0 ppm)	4 h/day, 5 day per week, 7 weeks, then 7 h/day, 5 days per week, 97 weeks	6 months	12/156	1/148
		- / 60[b]	0 mg/m^3 (0 ppm)				
		- / 54[b]	400 mg/m^3 (100 ppm)				
		62 / 61	400 mg/m^3 (100 ppm)			10/61	4/61
		60 / 60	400 mg/m^2 (100 ppm)	4 h/day, 5 days per week, 7 weeks, then 7 h/day, 5 days per week, 8 weeks	6 months	8/59	2/60

Table 10 (contd).

Rat, CD [118, 119]	inhalation	36	0 mg/m^3 (0 ppm)	6 h/day, 5 days per week,	none
		36	220 mg/m^3 (55 ppm)		none
Rat, CD [79]	inhalation			6h/day, 5 days per week for:	52 weeks
		4	0 mg/m^3 (0 ppm)	1 month	
		8	0 mg/m^3 (0 ppm)	3 months	
		8	0 mg/m^3 (0ppm)	6 months	
		16	0 mg/m^3 (0 ppm)	10 months	
		4	220 mg/m^3 (55 ppm)	1 month	
		8	220 mg/m^3 (55ppm)	3 months	
		8	220 mg/m^3 (55 ppm)	6 months	
		16	220 mg/m^3 (55 ppm)	10 months	
Rat, Sprague-Dawley [179, 180] [134, 178]	inhalation	86	0 mg/m^3 (0 ppm)	6 h/day, 5 days per week, 18 months	6 months
		86	40 mg/m^3 (10 ppm) first 5 weeks, then 100 mg/m^3 (25 ppm)		
		86	160 mg/m^3 (40 ppm) first 5 weeks, then 300 mg/m^3 (75 ppm)		

Table 10 (contd).

Species/strain (Reference)	Route (Vehicle)	Number of animals in each group male / female	Dose	Duration of administration	Post-exposure period	Result male	Result female
Rat, Wistar [229]	inhalation	30 / 30 51 / 23	0 mg/m^3 (0 ppm) 800 mg/m^3 (200 ppm) first 5 months, 400 mg/m^3 (100 ppm) subsequently	4 h/day, 5 days per week, for 12 months	to spontaneous death or moribund state	-	-
Rat, Sprague-Dawley [229]	inhalation	30 / 30 16 / 16 30 / 30	0 mg/m^3 (0 ppm) 300 mg/m^3 (75 ppm) 400 mg/m^3 (100 ppm)	4 h/day, 5 days per week, 12 months	to spontaneous death or moribund state (22 - 24 months)	only gross pathology performed	
Mouse, Swiss [139,141]	inhalation	190 / 190 30 / 30 150 / 150 30 / 30	0 mg/m^3 (0 ppm) 40 mg/m^3 (10 ppm) 100 mg/m^3 (25 ppm) 200 mg/m^3 (50 ppm)	4 h/day, 5 days per week, 52 weeks 4 h/day, 4 days^c	up to 121 weeks to spontaneous death	*Kidney adeno-carcinomas* 0/120 0/24 28/119 2/18	0/155 0/26 1/138 0/14

Table 10 (contd).

Mouse (Swiss) (contd). [139, 141]		Mammary gland adenomas	
	0 mg/m³ (0 ppm)	1/180	3/187
	40 mg/m³ (10 ppm)	0/30	6/30
	100 mg/m³ (25 ppm)	1/148	16/148
	200 mg/m³ (50 ppm)	0/52	6/54
		Lung (mainly adenomas)	
	0 mg/m³ (0 ppm)	6/154	7/178
	40 mg/m³ (10 ppm)	6/28	3/30
	100 mg/m³ (25 ppm)	23/141	12/147
	200 mg/m³ (50 ppm)	4/51	6/59
		Tumours of the mammary gland and lung were not dose-dependent	

Table 10 (contd).

Species/strain (Reference)	Route (Vehicle)	Number of animals in each group		Dose	Duration of administration	Post-exposure period	Result	
		male	female				male	female
Mouse, CD-1 [118, 119]	inhalation	36 36	36 36	0 mg/m^3 (0 ppm) 220 mg/m^3 (55 ppm)	6 h/day, 5 days per week, 52 weeks	none none	- Incidence of hepatic haemangiosarcoma and possibly bronchiolo-alveolar adenoma increased, but this is not thought to have been induced by vinylidene chloride [79]	-
Mouse, CD-1 [79]	inhalation	16 16 28 8 8 12	16 16 28 8 8 12	0 mg/m^3 (0 ppm) 0 mg/m^3 (0 ppm) 0 mg/m^3 (0 ppm) 220 mg/m^3 (55 ppm) 220 mg/m^3 (55 ppm) 220 mg/m^3 (55 ppm)	6 h/day, 5 days per week, for: 1 month 3 months 6 months 1 month 3 months 6 months	52 weeks	- - - - - -	- - - - - -

Table 10 (contd).

						to spontaneous death
Chinese Hamster [139, 141]	inhalation	18 30	17 30	0 mg/m³ (0 ppm) 100 mg/m³ (25 ppm)	4 h/day, 4 - 5 days per week, for 52 weeks	- - - -
Rat, Sprague-Dawley [179, 180] [177]	oral (drinking-water)	80	80	0 mg/litre (0 ppm)	daily for 24 months	none
		48	48	50 mg/litre (50 ppm) (M = 7 mg/kgbw) (F = 9 mg/kgbw)		none -
		48	48	100 mg/litre (100 ppm) (M = 10 mg/kgbw) (F = 14 mg/kgbw)		none -
		48	48	200 mg/litre (200 ppm) (M = 20 mg/kgbw) (F = 30 mg/kgbw)		none -

Table 10 (contd).

Species/strain (Reference)	Route (Vehicle)	Number of animals in each group		Dose	Duration of administration	Post-exposure period	Result	
		male	female				male	female
Rat, Sprague-Dawley [139, 141]	gavage (olive oil)	100	100	olive oil	daily 4 - 5 days/ week, for 52 weeks	to spontaneous death		
		82	77	(0 mg/kgbw)			-	-
		50	50	0.5 mg/kgbw			-	-
		50	50	5 mg/kgbw			-	-
		50	50	10 mg/kgbw			-	-
		50	50	20 mg/kgbw			-	-
Mouse, Swiss Ha: ICR; [227]	dermal (in 0.2 ml acetone)	100		0 mg	3 ×/week to spontaneous death or moribund state	none		
		30		0.1 ml acetone		none		
		30		40 mg/mouse		none		
		30		121 mg/mouse		none		
Mouse, Swiss Ha: ICR; [227]	subcutaneous (in 0.05 ml trioctanoin)	100		0 mg	once per week 649 days	none		
		30		0.05 ml water	636 days	none		
		30		0.05 ml trioctanoin	631 days	none	-	-
		30		2 mg/mouse	548 days	none	-	-

Table 10 (contd).

Species, strain; Ref.	Type of test	No. animals	Dose	Treatment schedule	Controls	Results
Mouse, Swiss Ha: ICR; [227]	dermal (initiation test on the skin)	30	121 mg/mouse then 5 mg PMA[d] per animal	once, to spontaneous death or moribund state; PMA 3 ×/week	none	8/30 papillomas 1/30 skin carcinoma

[a] Modified from: ECETOC [45].
[b] Only 2 treatments, because of the high toxicity.
[c] Pregnant females.
[d] Only 4 treatments, because of the high toxicity and mortality.
[e] PMA = phorbol myristate acetate.

9. EFFECTS ON HUMAN BEINGS

9.1 Single and Short-term Exposures

According to Gibbs & Wessling, [59], exposure to a high concentration of vinylidene chloride, e.g., 16 000 mg/m^3 (4000 ppm), rapidly causes intoxication that can lead to unconsciousness. The anaesthetic effects from short-term exposure are short-lived. At unspecified sub-anaesthetic doses, prolonged exposure and repeated short-term exposures may produce kidney and liver damage [221].

Some adverse effects associated with vinylidene chloride exposure have been attributed to contaminants or to the stabilizer (p-methoxyphenol). Henschler et al. [74] reported the occurrence of persistent cranial nerve disorders in two individuals who had attempted to clean out tanks that had contained vinylidene chloride co-polymers. The chemical responsible for this effect appeared, however, to be a contaminant of vinylidene chloride (either mono- or dichloroacetylene). Chivers [29] reported the incidence of leukoderma in two subjects following skin contamination with p-methoxyphenol. The irritant effect of vinylidene chloride [84, 192] on the eye, upper respiratory tract (at levels as low as 100 mg/m^3 i.e., 25 ppm) [192], and skin may be at least partially due to the stabilizer p-methoxyphenol and, in the case of the study by Rylova [192], other impurities. Dermatitis was reported in an individual whose skin was directly exposed to Saran film (vinylidene chloride/vinyl chloride co-polymer in the absence of a stabilizer) [160].

9.2 Long-Term Exposure

A quantitative risk estimate based on the best available set of data (mouse-kidney adenocarcinoma) from the animal tumour assays, using a non-threshold mathematical model, linear at low doses, provides an estimate of an upper limit of human risk [225]. The true risk is not likely to be greater than this estimate and may be lower. The upper limit for human risk thus estimated was 5.0×10^{-5} for a continuous lifetime exposure to 1µg/m^3 in air and 3.3×10^{-5}

for ingestion of drinking-water containing 1μg/litre. However, in the light of the discussion in section 8.6.4, the limited evidence for carcinogenicity in animal models is not sufficient to reach a firm conclusion on the carcinogenic risk of vinylidene chloride for human beings.

Interpretation of epidemiological studies on the effects of vinylidene chloride in human beings has been confounded by concomitant exposure to vinyl chloride. A mortality study on 629 workers exposed to vinylidene chloride, for 6–10 h/day, 42 h/per week, for various lengths of time in a vinylidene chloride production and polymerization plant in the Federal Republic of Germany was reported by Thiess et al. [219]. Individuals were exposed to an estimated (unmeasured) average plant concentration of 200 mg vinylidene chloride/m^3 (50 ppm) from 1955 to 1965 and subsequently to an average level of approximately 40 mg/m^3 (10 ppm) up to 1975, based on measurements of airborne contamination after 1975. All had also been exposed to vinyl chloride (measured as < 13 mg/m^3 (<5 ppm) since 1975) and acrylonitrile (measured as < 2 mg/m^3 (<1 ppm) since 1975). A 97% tracing was obtained for follow-up analysis of the majority (447) of the cohort that was exposed for more than 6 months. The incidence of exposure for >1 year in the remainder, was 36% and tracing for follow-up analysis was only 24%. The mortality rate of the cohort was compared with that of two populations of 180 000 (local) and 3 700 000 (regional) for the period 1969-75. The expected number of deaths was calculated by applying age-specific mortality rates to the person-years of observation of 7 age groups within the cohort. Statistical evaluation was based on the Poisson distribution. The distribution of deaths according to age and decade (total 39 deaths) indicated that workers in the exposure groups did not have an elevated mortality rate (total 57 and 36 expected from the data of the two reference populations). The expected numbers of deaths resulting from cancers, infectious diseases, cardiovascular diseases, other natural causes, and external causes were compared with the observed incidence.

Although the number of deaths from cardiovascular diseases in general was not different from that expected, a peculiar distribution of deaths caused by cerebral haemorrhage in the young age groups deserves mention. The occurrence of several deaths attributable to cerebral haemorrhage, cerebral sclerosis/apoplexia, and acute coronary failure in age-groups below 50 years was beyond chance (P-values far below 0.05). But this study did not verify the validity of diagnoses on death certificates and adequately designed studies are needed to ascertain this part of the mortality findings.

Five deaths (out of 39) through suicide compares with 2.5–3.0 expected. This cause of death does not rely on diagnostic validity and indicates the need for further investigations, because suicide may relate to mental depression. Bronchial carcinomas were seen in 5 individuals compared with expected numbers of 3.9 and 2.2 from the data on the two control populations. It was noted that 3 of the subjects with bronchial carcinoma were heavy smokers, the remaining 2 cases (observed at age 37) were clearly in excess of the expected incidence in the age-group below 40 (0.08 and 0.07 for the 2 reference populations, $P = 0.003$). The incidence of oesophageal cancer was within the range of age-specific expectation for the larger (district) control population but not for the smaller city population. The authors concluded that the overall malignant tumour incidence was not statistically different from the expected rate.

More detailed information was provided in a follow-up investigation of this exposed population (535 persons exposed for more than 6 months) [110]. In this extended analysis with an estimated average exposure in the years before 1965 of 200 mg/m^3 (50 ppm), the observed total number of deaths (48) was significantly greater than that expected from the reference populations (43.2–46.5) due to a greater incidence of cardiovascular disease (20 observed deaths versus about 15 expected). Eleven deaths from myocardial infarction were statistically significantly in excess of the 6.8 expected. The number of malignant tumours was 12 compared with 9.8 expected and this was reflected in the incidence of bronchial carcinomas (6 compared with 2.68–2.96 expected). In comparison with internal reference groups not exposed to vinylidene chloride, the cancer deaths were statistically in excess (3 of the lung-cancer cases were aged under 50). However, this statistically increased incidence was not considered to be related to vinylidene chloride exposure since, in 2 cases, exposure was limited to 2 years duration. The interpretation of the epidemiological study is hampered by a low cohort number, while co-exposure to other chemicals, such as vinyl chloride, was only considered in part by the inclusion of internal reference populations.

In a further epidemiological study [240], employees had been exposed to different extents to a range of substances in synthetic chemical plants. These investigators combined detailed work histories of 4806 individuals with exposure ratings for each of 19 chemicals during each calendar year from 1942 to 1973. After construction of a serially additive expected dose model, the authors tested whether vinylidene chloride was responsible for the observed excess risk of lung cancer in the cohort by using the one-sided t-test of the observed minus expected cumulative doses over all years and for ten or more years before death. No relationship was found between vinylidene chloride exposure and lung cancers.

The only epidemiological study of individuals exposed to vinylidene chloride where vinyl chloride was not used as a co-polymer (ethyl acrylate was the co-polymer) was carried out by Ott et al. [166]. Employees (138) were exposed to time-weighted average (TWA) concentrations ranging from 20 to 280 mg vinylidene chloride/m^3 (5 to 70 ppm) for a minimum of one year, within the period 1942-65. No association was found between exposure and mortality ascertained in 1974 among this low cohort number, when compared with US national statistics. Two employees suffered hepatic damage, but, in both cases, alcohol consumption was known to prevail. The size of the cohort having a long duration of exposure or a long latency period since initial exposure was small. No internal comparison was made, comparable to the approach by Klimish et al. [110]. Although the results of the epidemiological studies do not provide convincing evidence for an increased risk of cancer in human beings exposed to vinylidene chloride, it is not possible to conclude that there is no carcinogenic effect. It should be remembered that inadequate studies often tend to underestimate rather than to overestimate an association between exposure and cancer.

Schmitz et al. [198] assessed serum glutamic oxaloacetic transaminase, glutamic pyruvic transaminase, and γ-glutamyl transpeptidase in 133 human subjects exposed to vinylidene chloride, as a test for liver damage. Serum enzyme levels changed less in two comparison groups than in the exposed group but, according to Fisher's Exact Probability Test, the duration of exposure to vinylidene chloride did not influence the serum enzyme levels.

10. EVALUATION OF EFFECTS ON THE ENVIRONMENT AND HUMAN HEALTH RISKS

10.1 Evaluation of Effects on the Environment

As a result of volatilization, the atmosphere is the major environmental compartment for vinylidene chloride. The half-life of vinylidene chloride in the troposphere is expected to be approximately 2 days and therefore the compound is unlikely to participate in the depletion of the stratospheric ozone layer. Leaching and volatilization render soil and sediments minor compartments for vinylidene chloride in the environment and the level of this chlorinated hydrocarbon in the aqueous environment is also minimized by rapid volatilization. It is not known whether the degradation of compounds, such as trichloroethylene and perchloroethylene, which are often found in water, contributes in a significant manner to the levels of vinylidene chloride found in the environment.

The concentrations of vinylidene chloride found in environmental waters and the acute toxicity levels for fish and *Daphnia* indicate that acute toxic risks for the aquatic environment are minimal. Available data on long-term toxicity are insufficient to assess sublethal effects on any aquatic organisms residing near point sources of relatively high levels of vinylidene chloride contamination, such as contaminated ground water and municipal and industrial outfalls.

10.2 Evaluation of Human Health Risks

10.2.1 Levels of exposure

The general population is exposed to very low levels of vinylidene chloride. The maximum level reported in drinking-water is 20 µg/litre, though the average daily individual exposure of USA citizens via drinking-water has been estimated to be < 0.01 µg. The levels of vinylidene chloride in food are generally not detectable and levels above 10 µg/kg have not been reported. The levels in

Evaluation

food derived from aquatic organisms are not known, but are likely to be insignificant (section 10.1). Ambient air levels of vinylidene chloride have been reported of up to 52 $\mu g/m^3$ (at the perimeter of an industrial site). Median urban air concentrations in the USA of 20 ng/m^3 and 8.7 $\mu g/m^3$ have been reported for non-industrial and industrial-source areas, respectively.

Occupational exposure occurs particularly in production and polymerization processes. Respiration is the major route of uptake and the maximum recommended or regulated mean exposure limits over the period of a working day range from 8 to 500 mg/m^3 (or the lowest reliably detectable concentration) depending on the country. Short-term exposure limits range from 16 to 80 mg/m^3 and ceiling values range from 50 to 700 mg/m^3. Airborne levels of vinylidene chloride in the confined atmospheres to which workers in certain occupations are exposed have been found not to exceed 8 mg/m^3.

10.2.2 Acute effects

In human beings, inhalation of high concentrations of vinylidene chloride (very approximately, at or above the maximum olfactory threshold of 4000 mg/m^3) are likely to cause depression of the central nervous system and could lead to coma. On the basis of acute toxicity in animals, toxic effects of vinylidene chloride may occur in the liver, kidneys, or lungs at well below the minimum olfactory threshold of approximately 2000 mg/m^3. Vinylidene chloride exposure can lead to irritation of the eye, the upper respiratory tract (at 100 mg/m^3 in human beings (section 9.1), and the skin, and this is thought to be partially due to the stabilizer *p*-methoxyphenol.

In mice, which are more susceptible than rats to the hepatotoxic and renal toxic effects of vinylidene chloride, kidney damage was induced by exposure to as little as 40 mg vinylidene chloride/m^3 (10 ppm) for 6 h. Marked hepatotoxicity and renal toxicity were also seen in rats. After fasting, which exacerbated toxicity, exposure to vinylidene chloride at 600 mg/m^3 (150 ppm) and 800 mg/m^3 (200 ppm) for 6 h caused toxicity in rat liver and kidney, respectively. Studies on rats indicate that alcohol ingestion prior to exposure can enhance the metabolism and exacerbate the toxicity of vinylidene chloride. Acute toxicity is dependent on species, sex, strain, and the dietary status of animals. Species susceptibility is correlated with the activity of oxidative metabolism of vinylidene chloride in rats and mice. While it is not possible to predict whether the rat or the mouse provides the more suitable model for human beings, the activity of hepatic microsomal metabolism by human beings is quantitatively similar to that of the rat, a species of relatively low susceptibility. There is no evidence of a qualitative difference in the oxidative metabolism of vinylidene chloride in human beings and rodents.

It is apparent that the margin between the concentrations capable of producing toxicity in animals (40 mg/m^3 in mice) and the occupational exposure limit set by some countries may not be sufficient or may be non-existent.

10.2.3 Long-term effects and genotoxicity

Prolonged and repeated short-term exposures at sub-anaesthetic doses may produce kidney and liver damage. On the basis of long-term studies on animals, under conditions that simulated occupational exposure, hepatic changes were reported at an exposure level of 300 mg/m^3 (75 ppm) in rats. In mice, kidney and liver damage were seen at 100 mg/m^3 (25 ppm) and 200 mg/m^3 (50 ppm), respectively. There was considerable variation in the sensitivity to toxic effects observed in the different studies.

Vinylidene chloride does not appear to affect reproductive capacity or to pose an embryotoxic or teratogenic risk at dose levels below those required for maternal toxicity in animals, but this has not been studied in human beings. Embryo and fetal toxicity and fetal abnormalities were seen at levels producing maternal toxicity, as evidenced by reduced weight gain.

Vinylidene chloride is mutagenic for bacteria and yeast provided that a mammalian metabolic system is present. Some mammalian cells are also receptive to DNA damage and mutagenicity *in vitro*. Genotoxicity was not evident in the majority of *in vivo* studies on rodents, as measured by dominant lethality and cytogenetics, but aberrations in bone marrow cells of Chinese hamsters have been

Evaluation

reported. DNA binding and repair *in vivo* in rodents, though detectable, was minimal. The data on *in vivo* genetic studies therefore suggest some evidence for genetic toxicity, but, in the majority of studies, the effects were minimal or negative.

Several carcinogencity tests have been carried out on three species of experimental animals (mouse, rat, and hamster) using various routes of administration. Unfortunately, most of these studies suffered from severe limitations in design or conduct for carcinogenicity evaluation. No significant carcinogenic effects were observed in rats dosed orally. In adult rats exposed through inhalation, an increase in mammary tumours, which was not dose-related, was reported. A slight increase in leukaemia was observed, when rats were exposed both *in utero* and post-natally. These observations could not be evaluated. In one study on mice, increased incidence of kidney adenocarcinomas were observed in males at exposure levels of 200 and 100 mg/m^3 (50 and 25 ppm) but not at 40 and 0 mg/m^3 (10 and 0 ppm). In the same study, statistically increased incidences of lung tumours (mainly adenomas in both sexes) and mammary carcinomas (in females) were observed, but no dose-response relationships were found.

The kidney tumours may be related in some way to observed kidney cytotoxicity and it is possible that repeated kidney damage either leads directly to the carcinogenic response via a non-genotoxic mechanism or facilitates the expression of the genotoxic potential of metabolites in this particular species, sex, and organ. However, this conclusion is uncertain in the absence of adequate dose–response data on genetic effects *in vivo* and the findings that vinylidene chloride may have acted as an initiator in a two-stage skin assay in mice.

Epidemiological studies, while not providing any statistically significant evidence for an increased cancer risk from vinylidene chloride exposure under occupational conditions, are not adequate to permit a proper evaluation of the carcinogenic risk of vinylidene chloride for human beings.

Although the evaluations of individual authors dismiss the finding of excess cancer deaths as a chance occurrence (due to small numbers and cohort sizes), the consistency of the higher than expected values is worth mentioning. In the two cohort studies reported, lung cancer was observed in 7 cases, whereas 3.16 deaths would have been expected. The result cannot be dismissed, but co-existent exposure to vinyl chloride (in one study) has to be borne in mind. Since the cohorts were identified according to their exposure to vinylidene chloride, it may be impossible to exclude additional confounding exposures.

The morbidity findings reported (including one case of testicular carcinoma) have some informatory value. The interpretation by the authors that higher liver morbidity was related to the alcohol consumption of the individuals is invalid, since the alcohol intake by all members of the study (not only that of identified cases) was not assessed.

11. RECOMMENDATIONS

11.1 Recommendations for future work

There is a need for better estimates of the global annual production of vinylidene chloride and of the amounts of vinylidene chloride entering the environment from all sources, whether arising from the release of vinylidene chloride as such or from the degradation of other chemical products.

The predicted environmental fate is based on little experimental evidence. Information is required on rates of degradation and on transformation products in the air, soil, water, and sediment, and metabolism in representative non-mammalian species.

Long-term toxicity studies investigating a variety of pathological endpoints should be carried out on representative aquatic species (fish, crustacea, and molluscs).

Thresholds for, and mechanisms of, toxic effects from short- and long-term exposure to vinylidene chloride need to be defined more accurately in animals and human beings, as a basis for establishing safe levels of exposure.

More exhaustive use should be made of existing data on carcinogenicity. If further carcinogenicity studies are carried out, they should be conducted according to an accepted lifetime bioassay protocol specifically designed to cater for the particular properties of vinylidene chloride. Such studies should take into consideration the short half-life of the chemical in the body, the importance of age at onset of exposure, the daily exposure duration, and other relevant information that might be related to determining the dosing regimen. Species and strains of animals for testing need to be carefully selected. Toxicity data as well as metabolic and pharmacokinetic data for these animals would also be extremely useful.

Epidemiological studies are needed to enable an assessment to be made of the effects of exposure to vinylidene chloride (including prolonged low-level exposure) on human populations. Thus, long-term follow-up studies on morbidity and mortality on whole, unselected populations exposed to vinylidene chloride should be conducted. Information on effects, such as premature cerebro-vascular disease and cancer, is particularly necessary and studies should take into account confounding factors, such as smoking and alcohol consumption (ideally on a case-referent basis).

To overcome the problem of small numbers in individual production sites, multicentre studies with pooling of data may provide a valuable approach in both ongoing and future investigations. Historical data should be used as a reference basis for comparison with results from ongoing investigations to enable an assessment to be made of the protective effects of regulatory action over recent years.

There is a need to compare the *in vivo/in vitro* pharmacokinetics and metabolism of vinylidene chloride, especially in the kidney, liver, and lungs, in experimental animals of different species and in human beings, in order to better understand the results obtained in *in vivo* toxicity studies. Parallel data are required on the potential genotoxicity of vinylidene chloride at the target site for carcinogenesis in different species, to examine the possible role of a genetic mechanism.

In the light of the neurotoxicological findings reported in this review, there is a need to investigate the role of modulator systems in the pathogenesis of vinylidene chloride intoxication.

The value of the use of a sulfydryl agent, such as *N*-acetylcysteine, in the treatment of vinylidene chloride poisoning in human beings should be investigated in experimental animal studies.

11.2 Personal Protection and Treatment of Poisoning

11.2.1 Personal protection

In industrial situations where short-term inhalation exposures above the recommended limits are possible, full face masks with filters for organic vapours should be used and, where necessary for emergency use, masks with air-line supply systems should be provided. Properly maintained protective clothing including safety goggles should be worn by those handling vinylidene chloride, to prevent contact with the body. A constant air flow should be maintained within industrial plants with adequate filtered vents at points where spills or leaks are likely to occur. The monitoring of vinylidene chloride emissions during distribution operations is recommended. In the event of a leak, the vinylidene chloride should be evaporated either directly in the case of small leaks, or by controlled evaporation using an expansion synthetic foam. Water spray curtains can be used to disperse the vapour from the foam.

11.2.2 Treatment of poisoning in human beings

In cases of over-exposure or ingestion, medical advice should be obtained. Because of the irritant properties of vinylidene chloride, particular attention should be given to the lungs, skin, and eyes. The functions of the heart, liver, kidney, and central nervous system should be monitored. Since the animal data have indicated that vinylidene chloride produces a marked increase in sensitivity to epinephrine-induced cardiac arrhythmias, this drug should be avoided. Severe hypotension may be treated by transfusion, with whole blood or plasma expanders. There is no known antidote.

A patient poisoned through inhalation of vinylidene chloride should be kept warm in a semi-prone position, in fresh air. The airway should be kept clear and oxygen should be administered, if the subject is in a stupor or coma. Artificial respiration should be provided, if necessary.

Following ingestion of vinylidene chloride, the mouth should be rinsed with water. Vomiting should not be induced, because of the risk of aspiration of vinylidene chloride into the larynx and lungs. Gastric lavage and/or the oral administration of activated charcoal or liquid paraffin may help to reduce the bioavailability of vinylidene chloride, if given within approximately 1 h of ingestion, and may prove of benefit up to 4 h after ingestion.

Eyes exposed to vinylidene chloride should be immediately irrigated with water for at least 15 minutes and medical advice should be sought.

In the case of dermal exposure, contaminated clothing should be removed and the affected area of skin washed with soap and water.

12. PREVIOUS EVALUATIONS BY INTERNATIONAL BODIES

Vinylidene chloride was evaluated by WHO in 1984 [244] in the *Guidelines for drinking-water quality*. It was concluded that:

> "Dichloroethenes have been detected in drinking-water, generally at levels less than 1 µg/litre. The isomers have not always been differentiated. 1,1-dichloroethene is the isomer that causes most concern because of evidence that it is carcinogenic in experimental animals. It is a chemical commonly used in the synthesis of various polymers; for example, food wrappers are often made of 1,1-dichloroethene co-polymers. 1,1-Dichloroethene produces mammary tumours in both mice and rats, and kidney adenocarcinomas in mice (13). It has also been shown to be mutagenic in the Ames assay. A linear multi-stage extrapolation model was applied to data concerning the incidence of kidney adenocarcinomas in Swiss mice in order to calculate the recommended guideline value of 0.3 µg/litre."

Vinylidene chloride was evaluated by IARC Working Groups in 1978 [85], 1985 [86], and 1987 [87]. In 1987, the following conclusions were reported:

> **"VINYLIDENE CHLORIDE (Group 3)**
>
> **"A. Evidence for carcinogenicity to humans (*inadequate*)**
>
> "In one epidemiological study of 138 US workers exposed to vinylidene chloride, no excess of cancer was found, but follow-up was incomplete, and nearly 40% of the workers had less than 15 years' latency since first exposures. In a study in the Federal Republic of Germany of 629 workers exposed to vinylidene chloride, seven deaths from cancer (five bronchial carcinomas) were reported; this number was not in excess of the expected

value. Two cases of bronchial carcinoma were found in workers, both of whom were 37 years old, whereas 0.07 were expected for persons aged 35–39 years. The limitations of these two studies do not permit assessment of carcinogenicity of the agent to humans. No specific association was found between exposure to vinylidene chloride and the excess of lung cancer noted previously in a US synthetic chemicals plant.

"B. Evidence for carcinogenicity to animals (*limited*)

"Vinylidene chloride was tested for carcinogenicity in mice and rats by oral administration and by inhalation, in mice by subcutaneous administration and by topical application, and in hamsters by inhalation. Studies in mice and rats by oral administration gave negative results. In inhalation studies, no treatment-related neoplasm was observed in rats or hamsters. In mice, a treatment-related increase in the incidence of kidney adenocarcinomas was observed in male mice, as were increases in the incidence of mammary carcinomas in females and of pulmonary adenomas in male and female mice. In skin-painting studies in female mice, vinylidene chloride showed activity as an initiator, but, in a study of repeated skin application, no skin tumour occurred. No tumour at the injection site was seen in mice given repeated subcutaneous administrations.

"C. Other relevant data

"No data were available on the genetic and related effects of vinylidene chloride in humans.

"Vinylidene chloride did not induce dominant lethal mutations in mice or rats and did not induce chromosomal aberrations in bone-marrow cells of rats treated *in vivo*; however, it induced unscheduled DNA synthesis in treated mice. It did not induce chromosomal aberrations or mutation in Chinese hamster cells *in vitro* but did induce unscheduled DNA synthesis in rat hepatocytes. Vinylidene chloride was mutagenic to plant cells and induced mutation and gene conversion in yeast. It was mutagenic to bacteria."

REFERENCES

1 ALTMAN, P.L. & DITTMER, D.S. (1966) *Environmental biology*, Bethesda, Maryland, Federation of American Societies for Experimental Biology, pp. 326-328.

2 ANDERSEN, M.E. & JENKINS, L.J., Jr (1977) Oral toxicity of 1,1-dichloroethylene in the rat: effects of sex, age and fasting. *Environ. Health Perspect.* **21**: 157-163.

3 ANDERSEN, M.E., JONES, R.A., & JENKINS, L.J., Jr (1977) Enhancement of 1,1- dichloroethylene toxicity by pretreatment of fasted male rats with 2,3-epoxy-propan-1-ol. *Drug Chem. Toxicol.*,**1**: 63-74.

4 ANDERSEN, M.E, JONES, R.A., & JENKINS, L.J., Jr (1978) The acute toxicity of single, oral doses of 1,1-dichloroethylene in the fasted, male rat: effect of induction and inhibition of microsomal enzyme activities on mortality. *Toxicol. appl. Pharmacol.*, **46**: 227-234.

5 ANDERSEN, M.E., FRENCH, J.E, GARGAS, M.L., JONES, R.A., & JENKINS, L.J., Jr (1979a) Saturable metabolism and the acute toxicity of 1,1-dichloroethene. *Toxicol. appl. Pharmacol.*, **47**: 385-393.

6 ANDERSEN, M.E., GARGAS, M.L., JONES, R.A., & JENKINS, L.J., Jr (1979b) The use of inhalation techniques to assess the kinetic constants of 1,1-dichloroethylene metabolism. *Toxicol. appl. Pharmacol.*, **47**: 395-409.

7 ANDERSEN, M.E., THOMAS, O.E., GARGAS, M.L., JONES, R.A., & JENKINS, L.J., Jr (1980) The significance of multiple detoxification pathways for reactive metabolites in the toxicity of 1,1- dichloroethylene. *Toxicol. appl. Pharmacol,* **52**: 422-432.

8 ANDERSON, D., HODGE, M.C.E., & PURCHASE, I.F.H. (1977) Dominant lethal studies with the halogenated olefins vinyl chloride and vinylidene dichloride in male CD-1 mice. *Environ. Health Perspect.*, **21**: 71-78.

9 ATRI, F.R. (1985) [Chlorinated compounds in the environment.] *Schriftenr. Ver. Wasser-Boden-Lufthyg.*, **60**: 309-317 (in German)

10 BADEN, J.M., BRINKENHOFF, M., WHARTON, R.S., HITT, B.A., SIMMON, V.F., & MAZZE, R.I. (1976) Mutagenicity of volatile anesthetics. *Anesthesiology*, **45**: 311-318.

11 BADEN, J.M., KELLEY, M., SIMMON, V.F., RICE, S.A., & MAZZE, R.I. (1978) Fluroxene mutagenicity. *Mutat. Res.*, **58**: 183-191.

12 BADEN, J.M., KELLEY, M., & MAZZE, R.I. (1982) Mutagenicity of experimental inhalational anesthetic agents: sevofluorane, synthane, dioxychlorane and dioxyfluorane. *Anesthesiology*, **56**: 462-463.

13 BARRIO-LAGE, G., PARSONS, F.Z., NASSAR, R.S. & LORENZO, P.A. (1986) Sequential dehalogenation of chlorinated ethenes. *Environ. Sci. Technol.*, **20**, 96-99.

14 BARTSCH, H., MALAVEILLE, C., MONTESANO, R., & TOMATIS, L. (1975) Tissue-mediated mutagenicity of vinylidene chloride and 2-chlorobutadiene in *Salmonella typhimurium*. *Nature (Lond.)*, **255**: 641-643.

15 BARTSCH, H., MALAVEILLE, C., BARBIN, A., & PLANCHE, G. (1979) Mutagenic and alkylating metabolites of halo-ethylenes, chloro- butadienes and dichlorobutenes produced by rodent or human liver tissues. Evidence for oxirane formation by P450-linked microsomal mono-oxygenases. *Arch. Toxicol.*, **41**: 249-277.

16 BATTELLE (1983) *Study of discharges of certain chloroethylenes into the aquatic environment and the best technical means for the reduction of water pollution from such discharges*, Geneva, Battelle Institute (Contract U/82/-176(537).

17 BELLAR, T.A., BUDDE, W.L., & EICHELBERGER, J.W. (1979) The identification and measurement of volatile organic compounds in aqueous environmental samples. In: *94th ACS Symposium Series on Monitoring of Toxic Substances*, Washington, DC, American Chemical Society, pp. 49-62.

18 BIRKEL, T.J., ROACH, J.A.G., & SPHON, J.A. (1977) Determination of vinylidene chloride in saran films by electron capture gas-solid chromatography and confirmation by mass spectrometry. *J. Assoc. Off. Anal. Chem.*, **60**: 1210-1213.

19 BRONZETTI, G., BAUER, C., CORSI, C., LEPORINI, C., NIERI, R., & DEL CARRATORE, R. (1981) Genetic activity of vinylidene chloride in yeast. *Mutat. Res.*, **89**: 179-185.

20 BROWN, S.L., CHAN, F.Y., JONES, J.L., LIU, D.H., MCCALEB, K.E, MILL, T., SAPIO, K.N., & SCHENDEL, D.E. (1975) *Research program on hazard priority ranking of priority chemicals. Phase II: Final Report* Menlo Park, California, Stanford Research Institute (NSF-RA-E-75-190A; NTIS PB-263-161).

21 BUCCAFUSCO, R.J., ELLS, S.J., & LEBLANC, G.A. (1981) Acute toxicity of priority pollutants to bluegill (*Lepomis macrochirus*). *Bull. environ. Contam. Toxicol.*, **26**: 446-452.

22 BUCKINGHAM, J., ed. (1982) *Dictionary of organic compounds*, 5th ed., New York, Chapman and Hall, Vol. 2, p. 1733.

23 CARLSON, G.P. & FULLER, G.C. (1972) Interaction of modifiers of hepatic microsomal drug metabolism and the inhalation toxicity of 1,1-dichloroethylene. *Res. Commun. chem. Pathol. Pharmacol.*, **4**: 553-560.

24 CARPENTER, C.P., SMYTH, H.F., Jr, & POZZANI, U.C. (1949) The assay of acute vapor toxicity and the grading and interpretation of results of 96 chemical compounds. *J. ind. Hyg. Toxicol.*, **31**: 343-346.

25 CEC (1988) *Draft proposal for a Council Directive on the approximation of the laws of the Member States relating to plastic materials and*

articles intended to come into contact with foodstuffs, Brussels, Commission of the European Communities, p. 43.

26. CERNA, M. & KYPENOVA, H. (1977) Mutagenic activity of chloroethylenes analysed by screening system tests. *Mutat. Res.*, **46**: 214-215.

27. CHIECO, P., MOSLEN, M.T., & REYNOLDS, E.S. (1981) Effect of administrative vehicle on oral 1,1-dichloroethylene toxicity. *Toxicol. appl. Pharmacol.*, **57**: 146-155.

28. CHIECO, P., MOSLEN, M.T., & REYNOLDS, E.S. (1982) Histochemical evidence that plasma and mitochondrial membranes are primary foci of hepatocellular injury caused by 1,1-dichloroethylene. *Lab. Invest.*, **46**: 413-421.

29. CHIVERS, C.P. (1972) Two cases of occupational leucoderma following contact with hydroquinone monomethyl ether. *Br. J. ind. Med.*, **29**: 105-107.

30. COLE, R.H., FREDERICK, R.E., HEALY, R.P., & ROLAN, R.G. (1984) Preliminary findings of the priority pollutant monitoring project of the nationwide urban runoff program. *J. Water Pollut. Control Fed.*, **56**: 898-908.

31. COMBA, M.E. & KAISER, K.L.E. (1983) Determination of volatile contaminants at the $ng.1^{-1}$ level in water by capillary gas chromatography with electron capture detection. *Int. J. environ. anal. Chem.*, **16**: 17-31.

32. COSTA, A.K. & IVANETICH, K.M. (1982) Vinylidene chloride: its metabolism by hepatic microsomal cytochrome P-450 *in vitro*. *Biochem. Pharmacol.*, **31**: 2083-2092.

33. COSTA, A.K. & IVANETICH, K.M. (1984) Chlorinated ethylenes: their metabolism and effect on DNA repair in rat hepatocytes. *Carcinogenesis*, **5**: 1629-1636.

34. CUPITT, L.T. (1980) *Fate of toxic and hazardous materials in the air*, Washington, DC, US Environmental Protection Agency (EPA 600/83-80-084; PB 80-221948).

35. DALLAS, C.E., WEIR, F.W., FELDMAN, S., PUTCHA, L., & BRUCKNER, J.V. (1983) The uptake and disposition of 1,1-dichloroethylene in rats during inhalation exposure. *Toxicol. appl. Pharmacol.*, **68**: 140-151.

36. DAWSON, G.W., JENNINGS, A.L., DROZDOWSKI, D., & RIDER, E. (1975/77) The acute toxicity of 47 industrial chemicals to fresh and saltwater fishes. *J. hazard. Mater.*, **1**: 303-318.

37. DELEON, I.R., MABERRY, M.A., OVERTON, E.B., RASCHKE, C.K., REMELE, P.C., STEELE, C.F., WARREN, V.L., & LASETER, J.L. (1980) Rapid gas chromatographic method for the determination of volatile and semivolatile organochlorine compounds in soil and chemical waste disposal site samples. *J. chromatogr. Sci.*, **18**: 85-88.

References

38 DEMERTZIS, P.G., KONTOMINAS, M.G., & GILBERT, S.G. (1987) Gas chromatographic determination of sorption isotherms of vinylidene chloride n vinylidene chloride copolymers. *J.Food. Sci.*, **52**(3): 747- 750.

39 DILL, D.C., MCCARTY, W.M., ALEXANDER, H.C., & BARTLETT, E.A. (1980) *Toxicity of 1,1-dichloroethylene (vinylidene chloride) to aquatic organisms*, Midland, Michigan, Dow Chemical Company (PB 81-111098).

40 DILLING, W.L. (1977) Interphase transfer processes. II. Evaporation rates of chloromethanes, ethanes, ethylenes, propanes and propylenes from dilute aqueous solution. Comparison with theoretical predictions. *Environ. Sci. Technol.*, **11**: 405-409.

41 DOW (1988) *Migration of vinylidene chloride monomer into food simulating solvents from various vinylidene chloride copolymers. Report*, Midland, Michigan, Dow Chemical Company, p.6.

42 DOWD, R.M. (1985) EPA drinking-water proposals: round one. *Environ. Sci. Technol.*, **19**: 1156.

43 DREVON, C. & KUROKI, T. (1979) Mutagenicity of vinyl chloride, vinylidene chloride and chloroprene in V79 Chinese hamster cells. *Mutat. Res.*, **67**: 173-182.

44 EASLEY, D.M., KLEOPFER, R.D., & CARASEA, A.M. (1981) Gas chromatographic-mass spectrometric determination of volatile organic compounds in fish. *J. Assoc. Off. Anal. Chem.*, **64**: 653-656.

45 ECETOC (1985) Joint Assessment of Commodity Chemicals No.5:, *vinylidene chloride*, Brussels, European Chemical Industry Ecology and Toxicology Centre., 54 pp.

46 EISENREICH, S.J., LOONEY, B.B., & THORNTON, J.D. (1981) Airborne organic contaminants in the great lakes ecosystem. *Environ. Sci. Technol.*, **15**: 30-38.

47 EUROCOP-COST (1976) *Analysis of organic micropollutants in water*, Luxembourg, Commission of the European Communities (Cost Project 64b; EUCO/MDV/73/76, XII/476/76).

48 FERRARIO, J.B., LAWLER, G.C., DELEON, I.R., & LASETER, J.L. (1985) Volatile organic pollutants in biota and sediments of Lake Pontchartrain. *Bull. environ. Contam. Toxicol.* **34**: 246-255.

49 FILSER, J.G. & BOLT, H.M. (1979) Pharmacokinetics of halogenated ethylenes in rats. *Arch. Toxicol.*, **42**: 123-136.

50 FOERST, D. (1979) A sampling and analytical method for vinylidene chloride in air. *Am. Ind. Hyg. Assoc. J.*, **40**: 888-893.

51 FOGEL, M.M., TADDEO, A.R., & FOGEL, S. (1986) Biodegradation of chlorinated ethenes by a methane-utilizing mixed culture. *Appl. environ. Microbiol.*, **51**: 720-724.

52 FORKERT, P.G. & REYNOLDS, E.S. (1982) 1,1-dichloroethylene-induced pulmonary injury. *Exp. lung Res.*, **3**: 57-68.

53 FORKERT, P.G., FORKERT, L., FAROOQUI, M., & REYNOLDS, E.S. (1985) Lung injury and repair: DNA synthesis following 1,1-dichloroethylene. *Toxicology*, **36**: 199-214.

54 FORKERT, P.G., HOFLEY, M., & RACZ, W.J. (1986a) Metabolic activation of 1,1-dichloroethylene by mouse lung and liver microsomes. *Can. J. Physiol. Pharmacol.*, **65**: 1496-1499.

55 FORKERT, P.G., STRINGER, V., & RACZ, W.J. (1986b) Effects of administration of metabolic inducers and inhibitors on pulmonary toxicity and covalent binding by 1,1-dichloroethylene in CD-1 mice. *Exp. mol. Pathol.*, **45**: 44-58.

56 FORKERT, P.G., STRINGER, S., & TROUGHTON, K.M. (1986c) Pulmonary toxicity of 1,1-dichloroethylene correlation of early changes with covalent binding. *Can. J. Physiol. Pharmacol.*, **64**: 112-121.

57 GAGE, J.C. (1970) The subacute inhalation toxicity of 109 industrial chemicals. *Br. J. ind. Med.*, **27**: 1-18.

58 GAY, B.W., HANST, P.L., BUFALINI, J.J., & NOONAN, R.C. (1976) Atmospheric oxidation of chlorinated ethylenes. *Environ. Sci. Technol.*, **10**: 58-67.

59 GIBBS, D.S. & WESSLING, R.A. (1983) Vinylidene chloride and polyvinylidene chloride. In: Mark, H.F., Othmer, D.F., Overberger, C.G., & Seaborg, G.T., ed. *Kirk-Othmer encyclopedia of chemical technology*, 3rd ed., New York, John Wiley and Sons, Vol. 23, pp. 764- 798.

60 GILBERT, J., SHEPHERD, M.J., STARTIN, J.R., & MCWEENY, D.J. (1980) Gas chromatographic determination of vinylidene chloride monomer in packaging films and in foods. *J. Chromatogr.*, **197**: 71-78.

61 GLISSON, B.T., CRAFT, B.F., NELSON, J.H., & MEUZELAAR, H.L.C. (1986) Production of vinylidene chloride from the thermal decomposition of methyl chloroform. *Am. Ind. Hyg. Assoc. J.*, **47**: 427-435.

62 GOING, J.E. & SPIGARELLI, J. (1977) *Environmental monitoring near industrial sites - vinylidene chloride*, Washington, DC, US Environmental Protection Agency (EPA 560/6-77-026; NTIS PB- 273358).

63 GRASSELLI, J.R. & RITCHEY, W.M., ed. (1975) CRC *Atlas of spectral data and physical constraints for organic compounds*, Cleveland, Ohio, CRC Press, Vol. 3.

64 GREIM, H., BONSE, G., RADWAN, Z., REICHERT, D., & HENSCHLER, D. (1975) Mutagenicity *in vitro* and potential carcinogenicity of chlorinated ethylenes as a function of metabolic oxirane formation. *Biochem. Pharmacol.*, **24**: 2013-2017.

65 GRIMSRUD, E.P. & RASMUSSEN, R.A. (1975) Survey and analysis of halocarbons in the atmosphere by gas chromatography-mass spectroscopy. *Atmos. Environ.*, **9**: 1014-1017.

66 GRONSBERG, E.S. (1975) [Determination of vinylidene chloride in the air.] *Gig. i Sanit.*, **7**: 77-79 (in Russian).

67 GUILLEMIN, C.L., MARTINEZ, R., & THIAULT, S. (1979) Steam-modified gas-solid chromatography: a complementary technique for organic pollutant survey. *J. chromatogr. Sci.*, **17**: 677-681.

68 HARKOV, R., KEBBEKUS, B., BOZZELLI, J.W., & LIOY, P.J. (1983) Measurement of selected volatile organic compounds at three locations in New Jersey during the summer season. *J. Air Pollut Control Assoc.*, **33.** (12); 1177-1183.

69 HARKOV, R., KEBBEKUS, B., BOZZELLI, J.W., LIOY, P.J., & DAISEY, J. (1984) Comparison of selected volatile organic compounds during the summer and winter at urban sites in New Jersey. *Sci. total Environ.*, **38**: 259-274.

70 HARMS, M.S., PETERSON, R.E., FUJIMOTO, J.M., & ERWIN, C.P. (1976) Increased "bile duct-pancreatic fluid" flow in chlorinated hydrocarbon-treated rats. *Toxicol. appl. Pharmacol.*, **35**: 41-49.

71 HAWKINS, W.E., OVERSTREET, R.M., WALKER, W.W., & MANNING, C.S. (1985) Tumour induction in several small fish species by classical carcinogens and related compounds. In: *Proceedings of the Fifth Conference on Water Chlorination (Chemical, Environmental Impact and Health Effects)*, pp. 429-438.

72 HEITMULLER, P.T., HOLLISTER, T.A., & PARRISH, P.R. (1981) Acute toxicity of 54 industrial chemicals to sheepshead minnows (*Cyprinodon variegatus*). *Bull. environ. Contam. Toxicol.*, **27**: 596- 604.

73 HENSCHLER, D. (1977) Metabolism and mutagenicity of halogenated olefins. A comparison of structure and activity. *Environ. Health Perspect.*, **21**: 61-64.

74 HENSCHLER, D., BROSER, F., & HOPF, H.C. (1970) ["Polyneuritis cranialis" caused by poisoning with chlorinated acetylenes in working with vinylidene chloride copolymers.] *Arch. Toxicol.*, **26**: 62-75 (in German).

75 HEWITT, W.R. & PLAA, G.L. (1983) Dose-dependent modification of 1,1-dichloroethylene toxicity by acetone. *Toxicol. Lett.*, **16**: 145-152.

76 HIATT, M.H. (1983) Determination of volatile organic compounds in fish samples by vacuum distillation and fused silica capillary gas chromatography/mass spectrometry. *Anal. Chem.*, **55**: 506-516.

77 HOFMANN, H.T. & PEH, J. (1976) [*Report on the test of vinylidene chloride for mutagenic effects in Chinese Hamsters after subacute inhalation,*] Ludwigshafen, BASF Aktiengesellschaft, 22 pp. (in German).

78 HOLLIFIELD, H.C. & MCNEAL, T. (1978) Gas-solid chromatographic determination of vinylidene chloride in saran film and three simulating solvents. *J. Assoc. Off. Anal. Chem.*, **61**: 537-544.

79 HONG, C.B., WINSTON, J.M., THORNBURG, L.P., LEE, C.C., & WOODS, J. S. (1981) Follow-up study on the carcinogenicity of vinyl chloride and vinylidene chloride in rats and mice: tumor incidence and mortality subsequent to exposure. *J. Toxicol. environ. Health*, **7**: 909-924.

80 HSE (1983) *Methods for the determination of hazardous substances 28: Chlorinated hydrocarbon solvent vapours in air*, London, Health and Safety Executive.

81 HSE (1985) *Toxicity Review 13: Vinylidene chloride*, London, Health and Safety Executive, 59 pp.

82 HUBERMAN, E., BARTSCH, H., & SACHS, L. (1975) Mutation induction in Chinese hamster V79 cells by two vinyl chloride metabolites, chloroethylene oxide and 2-chloroacetaldehyde. *Int. J. Cancer*, **16**: 639-644.

83 HULL, L.A., HISATSUNE, I.C., & HEICKLEN, J. (1973) The reaction of O_3 with CCl_2CH_2. *Can. J. Chem.*, **51**: 1504-1510.

84 HUSHON, J. & KORNREICH, M. (1978) *Air pollution assessment of vinylidene chloride*, Washington, DC, US Environmental Protection Agency (EPA 450/3-78-015) (Prepared by the Metrek Division of the Mitre Corporation, McLean, Virginia; Contract No. 68-02-1495).

85 IARC (1979) *Some monomers, plastics and synthetic elastomers, acrolein*, Lyons, International Agency for Research on Cancer, pp. 439-459 (IARC Monograph on the Evaluation of the Carcinogenic Risk of Chemicals to Humans, Vol.19).

86 IARC (1986) *Some chemicals used in plastics and elastomers: vinylidene chloride*, Lyons, International Agency for Research on Cancer, pp. 195-226 (IARC Monographs on the Evaluation of the Carcinogenic Risk of Chemicals to Humans, Vol. 39).

87 IARC (1987) *Overall evaluations of carcinogenicity: An updating of IARC Monographs Vols. 1 - 42*, Lyons, International Agency for Research on Cancer, pp. 376-377 (IARC Monographs on the Evaluation of Carcinogenic Risks to Humans, Supplement 7).

88 IRPTC (1988) *IRPTC Legal file*, Geneva, International Register of Potentially Toxic Chemicals, United Nations Environment Programme.

89 ISHIDATE, M., Jr, ed. (1983) *The data book of chromosomal tests* in vitro *on 587 chemical substances using a Chinese hamster fibroblast cell line (Chl cells)*, Tokyo, The Realize Inc., p. 582.

90 JACKSON, N.M. & CONOLLY, R.B. (1985) Acute nephrotoxicity of 1,1- dichloroethylene in the rat after inhalation exposure. *Toxicol. Lett.*, **29**: 191-199.

91 JAEGER, R.J. (1975) Vinyl chloride monomer: comments on its hepatotoxicity and interaction with 1,1-dichloroethylene. *Ann. N.Y. Acad. Sci.*, **246**: 150-151.

92 JAEGER, R.J. & MURPHY, S.D. (1973) Alterations of barbiturate action following 1,1-dichloroethylene, corticosterone or acrolein. *Arch. int. Pharmacodyn.*, **205**: 281-292.

93 JAEGER, R.J., CONOLLY, R.B., & MURPHY, S.D. (1973a) Diurnal variation of hepatic glutathione concentration and its correlation with

1,1-dichloroethylene inhalation toxicity in rats. *Res. Commun. chem. Pathol. Pharmacol.*, **6**: 465-471.

94 JAEGER, R.J., TRABULUS, M.J., & MURPHY, S.D. (1973b) Biochemical effects of 1,1-dichloroethylene in rats: dissociation of its hepatotoxicity from a lipoperoxidative mechanism. *Toxicol. appl. Pharmacol.*, **24**: 457-467.

95 JAEGER, R.J., TRABULUS, M.J., & MURPHY, S.D. (1973c) The interaction of adrenalectomy, partial adrenal replacement therapy, and starvation with hepatotoxicity and lethality of 1,1- dichloroethylene intoxication. *Toxicol. appl. Pharmacol.*, **25**: 491 (Abstract No. 133).

96 JAEGER, R.J., CONOLLY, R.B., & MURPHY, S.D. (1974) Effect of 18-hr fast and glutathione depletion on 1,1-dichloroethylene-induced hepatotoxicity and lethality in rats. *Exp. mol. Pathol.*, **20**: 187-198.

97 JAEGER, R.J., SHONER, L.G., & COFFMAN, L. (1977a) 1,1- Dichloroethylene hepatotoxicity: proposed mechanism of action and distribution and binding of ^{14}C radioactivity following inhalation exposure in rats. *Environ. Health Perspect.*, **21**: 113-119.

98 JAEGER, R.J., SZABO, S., & COFFMAN, L.J. (1977b) 1,1- Dichloroethylene hepatotoxicity. Effect of altered thyroid funtion and evidence for the subcellular site of injury. *J. Toxicol. environ. Health*, **3**: 545-555.

99 JENKINS, L.J., Jr & ANDERSEN, M.E. (1978) 1,1-Dichloroethylene nephrotoxicity in the rat. *Toxicol. appl. Pharmacol.*, **46**: 131-141.

100 JENKINS, L.J., Jr, TRABULUS, M.J., & MURPHY, S.D. (1972) Biochemical effects of 1,1-dichloroethylene in rats: comparison with carbon tetrachloride and 1,2-dichloroethylene. *Toxicol. appl. Pharmacol.*, **23**: 501-510.

101 JONES, B.K. & HATHWAY, D.E. (1978a) Tissue-mediated mutagenicity of vinylidene chloride in *Salmonella typhimurium* TA1535. *Cancer Lett.*, **5**: 1-6.

102 JONES, B.K. & HATHWAY, D.E. (1978b) The biological fate of vinylidene chloride in rats. *Chem.-biol. Interact.*, **20**: 27-41.

103 JONES, B.K. & HATHWAY, D.E. (1978c) Differences in metabolism of vinylidene chloride between mice and rats. *Br. J. Cancer*, **37**: 411- 417.

104 KAISER, K.L.E., COMBA, M.E., & HUNEAULT, H. (1983) Volatile halocarbon contaminants in the Niagara River and in Lake Ontario. *J. Great Lakes Res.*, **9**(2): 212-223.

105 KANZ, M.F. & REYNOLDS, E.S. (1986) Early effects of 1,1-dichloroethylene on canalicular and plasma membranes: ultrastructure and stereology. *Exp. mol. Pathol.*, **44**: 93-110.

106 KANZ, M.F., WHITEHEAD, R.F., FERGUSON, A.E., & MOSLEN, M.T. (1988) Potentiation of 1,1-dichloroethylene hepatotoxicity: comparative effects of hyperthyreodism and fasting. *Toxicol. appl. Pharmacol.*, **95**: 93-103.

107 KIEZEL, L., LISZKA, M., & RUTKOWSKI, M. (1975) [Gas chromatographic determination of trace impurities in distillates of vinyl chloride monomer.] Chem. Anal. (Warsaw), 20: 555-562 (in Polish).

108 KLIMISCH, J.H. & FREISBERG, K.O. (1979a) [Report on the determination of acute toxicity (LC_{50}) by inhalation of vinylidene chloride in Chinese striped hamsters (fasting) during a 4-hour exposure period.], Ludwigshafen, BASF Aktiengesellschaft, 11 pp (in German).

109 KLIMISCH, J.H. & FREISBERG, K.O. (1979b) [Report on the determination of acute toxicity (LC_{50}) by inhalation of vinylidene chloride in Chinese striped hamsters (fed) during a 4-hour exposure period.], Ludwigshafen, BASF Aktiengesellschaft, 14 pp (in German).

110 KLIMISCH, J. H., LINK, R., STOCKER, W.G., & THIESS, A.M. (1982) Investigation of the mortality of workers predominantly exposed to vinylidene chloride. In: *Proceedings of the Medichem Congress, Paris, 1982.*

111 KRAMER, C.G. & MUTCHLER, J.E. (1972) The correlation of clinical and environmental measurements for workers exposed to vinyl chloride. *Am. Ind. Hyg. Assoc. J.*, **33**: 19-30.

112 KRIJGSHELD, K.R. & GRAM, T.E. (1984) Selective induction of renal microsomal cytochrome P-450-linked monooxygenases by 1,1-dichloroethylene in mice. *Biochem. Pharmacol.*, **33**: 1951-1956.

113 KRIJGSHELD, K.R., LOWE, M.C, MIMNAUGH, E.G., TRUSH, M.A, GINSBURG, E., & GRAM, T.E. (1983) Lung-selective impairment of cytochrome P- 450-dependent monooxygenases and cellular injury by 1,1-dichloroethylene in mice. *Biochem. biophys. Res. Commun.*, **110**: 675-681.

114 LAIB, R.J., KELIN, K.P., KAUFMANN, I., & BOLT, H.M. (1981) [On the problem of carcinogenicity of vinylidene chloride (1,1-dichloroethylene).] In: [*Epidemiological approaches in occupational medicine*], Stuttgart, Gentner Verlag, pp. 277-281 (in German).

115 LAO, R.C., THOMAS, R.S., BASTIEN, P., HALMAN, R.A., & LOCKWOOD, J.A. (1982) Analysis of organic priority and non-priority pollutants in environmental samples by GC/MS/computer systems. *Pergamon Ser. environ. Sci.*, **7**: 107-118.

116 LAZAREV, N.V., ed. (1960) [Vinylidene chloride.] In: [*Harmful substances in industry,*] Leningrad, Chemia, pp. 215-216 (in Russian).

117 LEBLANC, G.A. (1980) Acute toxicity of priority pollutants to water flea (*Daphnia magna*). *Bull. environ. Contam. Toxicol.*, **24**: 684-691.

118 LEE, C.C., BHANDARI, J.C., WINSTON, J.M., HOUSE, W.B., PETERS, P.J., DIXON, R.L., & WOODS, J.S. (1977) Inhalation toxicity of vinyl chloride and vinylidene chloride. *Environ. Health Perspect.*, **21**: 25- 32.

119 LEE, C.C., BHANDARI, J.C., WINSTON, J.M., HOUSE, W.B., DIXON, R.L., & WOODS, J.S. (1978) Carcinogenicity of vinyl chloride and vinylidene chloride. *J. Toxicol. environ. Health*, **4**: 15-30.

References

120 LEIBMAN, K.C. & ORTIZ, E. (1977) Metabolism of halogenated ethylenes. *Environ. Health Perspect.*, **21**: 91-97.

121 LESAGE, S., PRIDDLE, M.W., & JACKSON, R.E. (1988) *Organic contaminants in ground water at the Gloucester landfill.* Report, National Water Research Institute, Burlington, Ontario, p.13.

122 LIEBLER, D.C. & GUENGERICH, F.P. (1983) Olefin oxidation by cytochrome P-450: evidence for group migration in catalytic intermediates formed with vinylidene chloride and trans-1-phenyl-1-butene. *Biochemistry*, **22**: 5482-5489.

123 LIEBLER, D.C., MEREDITH, M.J., & GUENGERICH, F.P. (1985) Formation of glutathione conjugates by reactive metabolites of vinylidene chloride in microsomes and isolated hepatocytes. *Cancer Res.*, **45**: 186-193.

124 LIEBLER, D.C., LATWESEN, D.G. & REEDER, T.C. (1988). S-(2- chloroacetyl) glutathione, a reactive glutathione thiol ester and a putative metabolite of 1,1-dichloroethylene. *Biochemistry*, **27**: 3652- 3657.

125 LIN, S.-N., FU, F.W.-Y., BRUCKNER, J.V., & FELDMAN, S. (1982) Quantitation of 1,1- and 1,2-dichloroethylene in body tissues by purge-and-trap gas chromatography. *J. Chromatogr.*, **244**: 311-320.

126 LONG, R.M. & MOORE, L. (1987) Cytosolic calcium after carbon tetrachloride, 1,1-dichloroethylene, and phenylephrine exposure. Studies in rat hepatocytes with phosphorylase a and quin 2. *Biochem. Pharmacol.*, **36**: 1215-122

127 MABEY, W.R., SMITH, J.H., PUDOLL, R.T., JOHNSON, H.L., MILL, T., CHOU, T.W., GATES, J., PARTRIDGE, I.W., & VANDENBURG, D. (1981) *Aquatic fate process. Data for organic priority pollutants,* Washington, DC, US Environmental Protection Agency (EPA 440/4-81-014).

128 MCCANN, J., SIMMON, V., STREITWIESER, D., & AMES, B.N. (1975) Mutagenicity of chloroacetaldehyde, a possible product of 1,2-dichloroethane (ethylene dichloride), chloroethanol (ethylene chlorohydrin), vinyl chloride and cyclo-phosphamide. *Proc. Natl Acad. Sci. (USA)*, **72**: 3190-3193.

129 MCCARROLL, N.E., CORTINA, T.A., ZITO, M.J., & FARROW, M.G. (1983) Evaluation of methylene chloride and vinylidene chloride in mutational assays. *Environ. Mutagen.*, **5**: 426-427.

130 MCDONALD, T.J., KENNICUTT, M.C., & BROOKS, J.M. (1988) Volatile organic compounds at a coastal Gulf of Mexico site. *Chemosphere*, **17**, 123-136.

131 MCKENNA, M.J., WATANABE, P.G., & GEHRING, P.J. (1977) Pharmacokinetics of vinylidene chloride in the rat. *Environ. Health Perspect.*, **21**: 99-105.

132 MCKENNA, M.J., ZEMPEL, J.A, MADRID, E.O., & GEHRING, P.J. (1978a) The pharmacokinetics of [^{14}C]vinylidene chloride in rats following inhalation exposure. *Toxicol. appl. Pharmacol.*, **45**: 599-610.

133 MCKENNA, M.J., ZEMPEL, J.A, MADRID, E.O., BRAUN, W.H., & GEHRING, P.J. (1978b) Metabolism and pharmacokinetic profile of vinylidene chloride in rats following oral administration. *Toxicol. appl. Pharmacol.*, **45**: 821-835.

134 MCKENNA, M.J., QUAST, J.F., YAKEL, H.O., BALMER, M.F., & RAMPY, L.W. (1982) *Vinylindene chloride: a chronic inhalation toxicity and carcinogenicity study in rats. Final Report*, Midland, Michigan, Dow Chemical, 100 pp.

135 MAFF (1980) *Survey of vinylidene chloride levels in food contact materials and in foods. Third Report of the Steering Group on Food Surveillance: Working Party on Vinylidene Chloride*, London, Ministry of Agriculture, Fisheries and Food, 23 pp (Food Surveillance Paper No. 3).

136 MALAVEILLE, C., BARTSCH, H., BARBIN, A., CAMUS, A.M., MONTESANO, R., CROISY, A., & JACQUIGNON, P. (1975) Mutagenicity of vinyl chloride, chloroethylene-oxide, chloroacetylaldehyde and chloroethanol. *Biochem. biophys. Res. Commun.*, **63**: 363-370.

137 MALAVEILLE, C., PLANCHE, G., & BARTSCH, H. (1977) Factors for efficiency of the *Salmonella* microsome, mutagenicity assay. *Chem.- biol. Interact.*, **17**: 129-136.

138 MALTONI, C. & PATELLA, V. (1983) Comparative acute toxicity of vinylidene chloride. The role of species, strain and sex. *Acta oncol.*,**4**: 239-256.

139 MALTONI, C., COTTI, G., MORISI, L., & CHIECO, P. (1977) Carcinogenicity biosassays of vinylidene chloride. Research plan and early results. *Med. Lav.*, **68**: 241-262.

140 MALTONI, C., CILIBERTI, A., & CARRETTI, D. (1982) Experimental contributions in identifying brain potential carcinogens in the petrochemical industry. *Ann. N.Y. Acad. Sci.*, **381**: 216-249.

141 MALTONI, C., COTTI, G., & CHIECO, P. (1984) Chronic toxicity and carcinogenicity bioassays of vinylidene chloride. *Acta oncol.*, **5**: 91- 146.

142 MALTONI, C., LEFEMINE, G., COTTI, G., CHIECO, P., & PATELLA, V. (1985) Experimental research on vinylidene chloride carcinogenesis. In: Maltoni, C. & Mehlinan, M.A., ed. *Archives of research in industrial carcinogenesis*, Princeton, New Jersey, Princeton Scientific Publishers, Vol. 3, p.95.

143 MASUDA, Y. & NAKAYAMA, N. (1983) Protective action of diethyldithiocarbamate and carbon disulfide against acute toxicities induced by 1,1-dichloroethylene in mice. *Toxicol. appl. Pharmacol.*, **71**: 42-53.

144 MOTEGI, S., UEDA, K., TANAKA, H., & OHTA, M. (1976) Determination of residual vinylidene chloride monomer in polyvinylidene chloride films used for fish jelly products. *Bull. Jpn. Soc. Sci. Fish.*, **42**: 1387-1394.

References

145 MOORE, L. (1980) Inhibition of liver microsome calcium pump by in vivo administration of CCl_4, $CHCl_3$ and 1,1-dichloroethylene (vinylidene chloride). *Biochem. Pharmacol.*, **29**: 2505-2511.

146 MORTELMANS, K., HAWORTH, S., LAWLOR, T., SPECK, W., TAINER, B., & ZEIGER, E. (1986) *Salmonella* mutagenicity tests *III*. Results from the testing of 270 chemicals, *Environ. Mutat.*, **8**, (Suppl. 7): 1-119.

147 MOSLEN, M.T. & REYNOLDS, E.S. (1985) Rapid, substrate-specific and dose-dependent deactivation of liver cytosolic glutathione S- transferases in vivo by 1,1-dichloro-ethylene.*Res. Commun. chem. Pathol. Pharmacol.*, **47**: 59-72.

148 MOSLEN, M.T., POISSON, L.R., & REYNOLDS, E.S. (1985) Cholestasis and increased biliary excretion of inulin in rats given 1,1- dichloroethylene. *Toxicology*, **34**: 201-209.

149 MURRAY, F.J., NITSCHKE, K.D., RAMPY, L.W., & SCHWETZ, B.A. (1979) Embryotoxicity and fetotoxicity of inhaled or ingested vinylidene chloride in rats and rabbits. *Toxicol. appl. Pharmacol.*, **49**: 189- 202.

150 NEUFELD, M.L., SITTENFIELD, M., WOLK, K.F., & BOYD, R.E. (1977) *Market input/output studies. Task 1: vinylidene chloride*, Washington, DC, US Environmental Protection Agency (EPA 560/6-77-003; NTIS PB-273-205) (Prepared by Auerbach Associates; Contract No. 68- 01-1996).

151 NITSCHKE, K.D, SMITH, F.A., QUAST, J.F., NORRIS, J.M., & SCHWETZ, B.A. (1983) A three-generation rat reproductive toxicity study of vinylidene chloride in the drinking water. *Fundam. appl. Toxicol.*, **3**: 75-79.

152 NORRIS, J.M. (1977) Toxicological and pharmacokinetic studies on inhaled and ingested vinylidene chloride in laboratory animals. In: *Proceedings of the Technical Association of the Pulp and Paper Industry (TAPPI) Paper Synthetics Conference, Chicago, Illinois, 1977*, Atlanta, Georgia, Technical Association of the Pulp and Paper Industry, pp. 45-50.

153 NORRIS, J.M. & REITZ, R.H. (1984) *Interpretative review of the animal toxicological, pharmacokinetic/metabolism, biomolecular and* in vitro *mutagenicity studies on vinylidene chloride and the significance of the findings for man*, Midland, Michigan, Dow Chemical Co., p. 24.

154 NTP (1982) *Carcinogenesis bioassay of vinylidene chloride (CAS No. 75-35-4) in F344 rats and B6C3F1 mice (gavage study)*, Research Triangle Park, North Carolina, National Toxicology Program (Technical Report Series No. 228; PB 82-258393).

155 OBLAS, D.W., DUGGER, D.L., & LIEBERMAN, S.I. (1980) The determination of organic species in the telephone central office ambient. *IEEE Trans. Compnents Hybrids Manuf. Technol.*, **CHMT-3** (1): 17-20.

156 OESCH, F., PROTIC-SABLJIC, M., FRIEDBERG, T., KLIMISCH, H.J., & GLATT, H.R. (1983) Vinylidene chloride: changes in drug metabolising enzyme, mutagenicity and relation to its targets for carcinogenesis. *Carcinogenesis*, **4**: 1031-1038.

157 OKINE, L.K.N. & GRAM, T.E. (1986a) Tissue distribution and covalent binding of [^{14}C]1,1-dichloroethylene in mice. In vivo and in vitro studies. Adv. exp. Med. Biol., **197**: 903-910.

158 OKINE, L.K.N. & GRAM, T.E. (1986b) In vitro studies on the metabolism and covalent binding of [^{14}C]1,1-dichloroethylene by mouse liver, kidney and lung. Biochem. Pharmacol., **35**: 2789-2795.

159 OKINE, L.K.N., GOOCHEE, J.M., & GRAM, T.E. (1985) Studies on the distribution and covalent binding of 1,1-dichloroethylene in the mouse.Effects of various pretreatments on covalent binding in vivo. Biochem. Pharmacol., **34**: 4051-4057.

160 OSBOURNE, R.A. (1964) Contact dermatitis caused by saran wrap. J. Am. Med. Assoc., **188**: 1159.

161 OTSON, R. (1987) Purgeable organics in Great Lakes raw and treated water. Int. J. Environ. anal. Chem., **31**: 41-53.

162 OTSON, R. & WILLIAMS, D.T. (1982) Headspace chromatographic determination of water pollutants. Anal. Chem., **54**: 942-946.

163 OTSON, R., WILLIAMS, D.T., & BIGGS, D.C. (1982a) Relationships between raw water quality, treatment and occurrence of organics in Canadian potable water. Bull. environ. Contam. Toxicol., **28**: 396- 403.

164 OTSON, R., WILLIAMS, D.T., & BOTHWELL, P.D. (1982b) Volatile organic compounds in water at thirty Canadian potable water treatment facilities. J. Assoc. Off. Anal. Chem., **65**: 1370-1374.

165 OTT, M.G., LANGNER, R.R., & HOLDER, B.B. (1975) Vinyl chloride exposure in a controlled industrial environment. A long-term mortality experience in 594 employees. Arch. environ. Health, **30**: 333-339.

166 OTT, M.G., FISHBECK, W.A, TOWNSEND, J.C., & SCHNEIDER, E.J. (1976) A health study of employees exposed to vinylidene chloride. J.. occup. Med., **18**: 735-738.

167 PARSONS, F., WOOD, P.R., & DEMARCO, J. (1984) Transformations of tetrochloroethene and trichloroethene in microcosms and groundwater. J. Am. Water Works Assoc., **February**: 56-59.

168 PATTERSON, J.W. & KODUKALA, P.S. (1981) Biodegradation of hazardous organic pollutants. CEP, **April**: 48-55.

169 PEARSON, C.R. & MCCONNELL, G. (1975) Chlorinated C_1 and C_2 hydrocarbons in the marine environment.Proc. R. Soc. Lond. Ser. B,**189**: 305-332.

170 PFAB, W., VON & MUCKE, G. (1977) [On the migration of selected monomers in foodstuffs and simulations.] Dtsch. Lebensm. Rundschau, **73**: 1-5 (in German).

171 PIET, G.J., SLINGERLAND, P., DE GRUNT, F.E., VAN DEN HEUVEL, M.P.M., & ZOETEMAN, B.C.J. (1978) Determination of very volatile halogenated organic compounds in water by means of direct head-space analysis. Anal. Lett., **A11**(5): 437-448.

172 PONOMARKOV, V. & TOMATIS, L. (1980) Long-term testing of vinylidene chloride and chloroprene for carcinogenicity in rats. *Oncology*, **37**: 136-141.

173 PRENDERGAST, J.A., JONES, R.A, JENKINS, L.J., Jr, & SIEGEL, J. (1967) Effects on experimental animals of long-term inhalation of trichloroethane, carbon tetrachloride, 1,1,1-trichloro-ethylene, dichlorodifluoromethane and 1,1-dichloroethylene. *Toxicol. appl. Pharmacol.*, **10**: 270-289.

174 PRICE, P.S. (1985) *Volatile organochlorine compounds (VOC) degradation. Technical Memorandum*, Washington, DC, US Environmental Protection Agency, p.19.

175 PUTCHA, L., BRUCKNER, J.V., D'SOUZA, R., DESAI, F., & FELDMAN, S. (1986) Toxicokinetics and bioavailability of oral and intravenous 1,1-dichloroethylene. *Fundam. appl. Toxicol.*, **6**: 240-250.

176 QUAST, J.F., HUMISTON, C.G., SCHWETZ, B.A., BALMER, M.F., RAMPY, L.W., NORRIS, J.M., & GEHRING, P.J. (1977) Results of 90-day toxicity study in rats given vinylidene chloride in their drinking water or exposed to VDC vapour by inhalation. *Toxicol. appl. Pharmacol.*, **4**: 187.

177 QUAST, J.F., HUMISTON, C.G., WADE, C.E., BALLARD, J., BEYER, J.E, SCHWETZ, R.W., & NORRIS, J.M. (1983) A chronic toxicity and oncogenicity study in rats and subchronic toxicity study in dogs on ingested vinylidene chloride. *Fundam. appl. Toxicol.*, **3**: 55-62.

178 QUAST, J.F., MCKENNA, M.J., RAMPY, L.W., & NORRIS, J.M. (1986) Chronic toxicity and oncogenicity study on inhaled vinylidene chloride in rats. *Fundam. appl. Toxicol.*, **6**: 105-144.

179 RAMPY, L.W., QUAST, J.F., HUMISTON, C.G., BALMER, M.F., & SCHWETZ, B.A. (1977) Interim results of two-year toxicological studies in rats of vinylidene chloride incorporated in the drinking water or administered by repeated inhalation. *Environ. Health Perspect.*, **21**: 33-43.

180 RAMPY, L.W., QUAST, J.F., HUMISTON, C.G., BALMER, M.F., & SCHWETZ, B.A. (1978) Results of two-year toxicological studies in rats of vinylidene chloride incorporated in the drinking water or administered by repeated inhalation. *Toxicol. appl. Pharmacol.*, **45**: 244-245.

181 RAMSTAD, T., NESTRICK, T.J., & PETERS, T.L. (1981) Applications of the purge-and-trap technique. *Am. Lab.*, **13**: 65-73.

182 RAY, P. & MOORE, L. (1982) 1,1-Dichloroethylene inhibition of liver microsomal calcium pump *in vitro*. *Arch. Biochem. Biophys.*, **218**: 26-30.

183 REICHERT, D., WERNER, H.W., & HENSCHLER, D. (1978) Role of liver glutathione in 1,1-dichloroethylene metabolism and hepatotoxicity in intact rats and isolated perfused rat liver. *Arch. Toxicol.*, **41**: 169-178.

184 REICHERT, D., WERNER, H.W., METZLER, M., & HENSCHLER, D. (1979) Molecular mechanism of 1,1-dichloroethylene toxicity: excreted

metabolites reveal different pathways of reactive intermediates. *Arch. Toxicol.*, **42**: 159-169.

185 REICHERT, D., SPENGLER, U., ROMEN, W., & HENSCHLER, D. (1984) Carcinogenicity of dichloroacetylene: an inhalation study. *Carcinogenesis*, **5**: 1411-1420.

186 REITZ, R.H., WATANABE, P.G., MCKENNA, M.J., QUAST, J.F., & GEHRING, P.J. (1980) Effects of vinylidene chloride on DNA synthesis and DNA repair in the rat and mouse: a comparative study with dimethylnitrosamine. *Toxicol. appl. Pharmacol.*, **52**: 357-370.

187 REKKER, R.F. (1977) The hydrophobic fragment constant, its derivation and application. A means of characterizing membrane systems. In: Nauta, W.Th. & Rekker, R.F., ed. *Pharmacochemistry library*, Amsterdam, Elsevier Scientific Publishers, Vol. 1.

188 REYNOLDS, E.S, MOSLEN, M.T., SZABO, S., JAEGER, R.J., & MURPHY, S.D. (1975) Hepatotoxicity of vinyl chloride and 1,1-dichloroethylene. Role of mixed function oxidase system. *Am. J. Pathol.*, **81**: 219-236.

189 REYNOLDS, E.S, MOSLEN, M.T., BOOR, P.J., & JAEGER, R.J. (1980) 1,1- Dichloroethylene hepatotoxicity. Time course of GSH changes and biochemical aberrations. *Am. J. Pathol.*,**101**: 331-344.

190 REYNOLDS, E.S., KANZ, M.F., CHIECO, P., & MOSLEN, M.T. (1984) 1,1- Dichloroethylene: an apoptotic hepatotoxin. *Environ. Health Perspect.*, **57**: 313-320.

191 RUSSELL, M.J. (1975) Analysis of air pollutants using sampling tubes and gas chromatography. *Environ. Sci. Technol.*, **9**: 1175-1178.

192 RYLOVA, M.L. (1953) [Toxicity of vinylidene chloride.] *Farmakol. Toksikol.*, **16**(1): 47-50 (in Russian).

193 SASAKI, M., SUGIMURA, K., YOSHIDA, M.A., & ABE, S. (1980) Cytogenetic effects of 60 chemicals on cultured human and Chinese hamster cells. *Kromosomo* II,**20**: 574-584.

194 SASSU, G.M, ZILIO-GRANDI, F., & CONTE, A. (1968) Gas chromatographic determination of impurities in vinyl chloride.J. *Chromatogr.*, **34**: 394-398.

195 SATO, A., NAKAJIMA, T., & KOYAMA, Y. (1980) Effects of chronic ethanol consumption on hepatic metabolism of aromatic and chlorinated hydrocarbons in rats. *Br. J. ind. Med.*, **37**: 382-386.

196 SAWADA, M., SOFUNI, T., & ISHIDATE, M., Jr (1987) Cytogenetic studies on 1,1-dichloroethylene and its two isomers in mammalian cells in vitro and in vivo. *Mutat. Res.*, **187**: 157-163.

197 SAX, N.I. (1984) *Dangerous properties of industrial materials*, 6th ed., New York, Van Nostrand Reinhold, p. 2730.

198 SCHMITZ, TH., THIESS, A.M., & PENNING, E. (1979) [Inquiry into morbidity among workers exposed to vinylidene chloride (VDC) and polyvinylidene chloride (PVDC).] In: [*Report on the Tenth Annual*

References

Meeting of the German Occupational Medicine Society together with the Federation of Industrial Employers Associations, Munster, 2-5 May, 1979,] Stuttgart, Gentner Verlag (in German).

199 SEVERS, L.W. & SKORY, L.K. (1975) Monitoring personnel exposure to vinyl chloride, vinylidene chloride and methyl chloride in an industrial work environment. *Am. Ind. Hyg. Assoc. J.*, **39**: 669-676.

200 SHACKELFORD, W.M. & KEITH, L.H. (1976) *Frequency of organic compounds identified in water*, Washington, DC, US Environmental Protection Agency, Office of Research and Development, Environmental Research Laboratory (EPA 600/4-76-062; PB-265-470).

201 SHELTON, L.G., HAMILTON, D.E., & FISACKERLY, R.H. (1971) Vinyl and vinylidene chloride. In: Leonard, E.C., ed. *Vinyl and diene monomers. Part 3*, New York, Wiley Interscience, pp. 1505-1289.

202 SHORT, R.D., MINOR, J.L., PETERS, P., WINSTON, J.M., FERGUSON, B., UNGER, T., SAWYER, M., & LEE, C.C. (1977a) *The developmental toxicity of vinylidene chloride inhaled by rats and mice during gestation*, Washington, DC, US Environmental Protection Agency (EPA 560/6-77-022; PB-281-713) (Prepared by Midwest Research International, Kansas City, Missouri).

203 SHORT, R.D., MINOR, J.L., WINSTON, J.M., & LEE, C.C. (1977b) A dominant lethal study in male rats after repeated exposures to vinyl chloride or vinylidene chloride. *J. Toxicol. environ. Health*, **3**: 965-968.

204 SHORT, R.D., WINSTON, J.M., MINOR, J.L., HONG, C.B., SEIFTER, J., & LEE, C.C. (1977c) Toxicity of vinylidene chloride in mice and rats and its alteration by various treatments. *J. Toxicol. environ. Health*, **3**: 913-921.

205 SIDHU, K.S. (1980) A gas-chromatographic method for the determination of vinylidene chloride in air. *J. anal. Toxicol.*, **4**: 266-268.

206 SIEGEL, J., JONES, R.A., COON, R.A., & LYON, J.P. (1971) Effects on experimental animals of acute, repeated and continuous inhalation exposures to dichloroacetylene mixtures. *Toxicol. appl. Pharmacol.*, **18**: 168-174.

207 SIEGERS, C.-P., YOUNES, M., & SCHMITT, G. (1979) Effects of dithiocarb and (+)-cyanidanol-3 on the hepatotoxicity and metabolism of vinylidene chloride in rats. *Toxicology*, **15**: 55-64.

208 SIEGERS, C.-P., HEIDBUCHEL, K., & YOUNES, M. (1983) Influence of alcohol, dithiocarb, or (+)-catechin on the hepatotoxicity and metabolism of vinylidene chloride in rats. *J. appl. Toxicol.*, **3**: 90-95.

209 SIEGERS, C.-P., HORN, W., & YOUNES, M. (1985a) Effect of hypoxia on the metabolism and hepatoxicity of carbon tetrachloride and vinylidene chloride in rats. *Acta pharmacol. toxicol.*, **56**: 81-86.

210 SIEGERS, C.-P., HORN, W., & YOUNES, M. (1985b) Effect of phorone-induced glutathione depletion on the metabolism and hepatotoxicity of carbon tetrachloride and vinylidene chloride. *J. appl. Toxicol.*, **5**: 352-356.

211 SILETCHNIK, L.M. & CARLSON, G.P. (1974) Cardiac sensitizing effects of 1,1-dichloroethylene: enhancement by phenobarbital pretreatment. Arch. int. Pharmacodyn., **210**: 359-364.

212 SINGH, H.B., SALAS, L.J., SMITH, A.J., & SHIGEISHI, M. (1981) Measurements of some potentially hazardous organic chemicals in urban environments. Atmos. Environ., **15**: 601-612.

213 SINGH, H.B., SALAS, L.J., & STILES, R.E. (1982) Distribution of selected gaseous organic mutagens and suspect carcinogens in ambient air. Environ. Sci. Technol., **16**: 872-880.

214 SPEIS, D.N. (1980) Determination of purgeable organics in sediments. Environ. Sci. Res., **16**: 201-206.

215 SWEGER, D.M. & TRAVIS, J.C. (1979) An application of infrared lasers to the selective detection of trace organic gases. Appl. Spectrosc., **33**: 46-51.

216 SZABO, S., JAEGER, R.J., MOSLEN, M.T., & REYNOLDS, E.S. (1977) Modification of 1,1-dichloroethylene hepatotoxicity by hypothyroidism. Toxicol. appl. Pharmacol., **42**: 367-376.

217 TABAK, H.H., QUAVE, S.A., MASHNI, C.I., & BARTH, E.F. (1981) Biodegradability studies with organic priority pollutant compounds. J. Water Pollut. Control Fed., **53**: 1503-1518.

218 TAN, S. & OKADA, T. (1979) Determination of residual vinylidene chloride monomer in polyvinylidene chloride. Hygienic studies on plastic containers and packages. III. J. Food Hyg. Soc. Jpn, **20**: 223-227.

219 THIESS, A.M., FRENTZEL-BEYME, R., & PENNING, E. (1979) Mortality study of vinylidene chloride exposed persons. In: Heim, C. & Kilian, D.J.., ed. *Proceedings of the 5th Medichem Congress, San Francisco, September 1977*, pp. 270-278.

220 THOMPSON, J.A, HO, B., & MASTOVICH, S.L. (1984) Reductive metabolism of 1,1,1,2-tetrachloroethane and related chloro-ethanes by rat liver microsomes. Chem-biol. Interact., **51**: 321-333.

221 TIERNEY, D.R., BLACKWOOD, T.R., & PIANA, M.R. (1979) *Status assessment of toxic chemicals: vinylidene chloride*, Cincinnati, Ohio, US Environmental Protection Agency (EPA 600/2-79-2100; PB 80- 146442).

222 TORKELSON, T.R. & ROWE, V.K. ed. (1982) Vinylidene chloride. In: Clayton, G.D. & Clayton, F.E., *Patty's industrial hygiene and toxicology*, 3rd ed., New York, John Wiley and Sons, pp. 3545-3550.

223 US EPA (1984a) Method 601. Guidelines establishing test procedures for the analysis of pollutants under the Clean Water Act (40 CFR 136). Purgeable halocarbons. Fed. Reg., **49**: 43261-43271.

224 US EPA (1984b) Method 1624, Revision B. Guidelines establishing test procedures for the analysis of pollutants under the Clean Water Act (40 CFR 136). Volatile organic compounds by isotope dilution GC/MS. Fed. Reg., **49**: 43407-43415.

References

225 US EPA (1985) *Health assessment document for vinylidene chloride*, Washington, DC, US Environmental Protection Agency, Office of Health and Environmental Assessment (EPA 600/8-83-031F).

226 US NIOSH (1987) *Manual of analytical methods*, 3rd ed., Cincinnati, Ohio, National Institute of Health and Human Services, pp.1-3 (Method 1015).

227 VAN DUUREN, B.L., GOLDSCHMIDT, B.M., LOEWENGART, G., SMITH, A.C., MELCHIONNE, S., SEIDMAN, I., & ROTH, D. (1979) Carcinogenicity of halogenated olefinic and aliphatic hydrocarbons in mice. *J. Natl Cancer Inst.*, **63**: 1433-1439.

228 VAN'T HOF, J. & SCHAIRER, L.A. (1982) *Tradescantia* assay system for gaseous mutagens. A report of the US Environmental Protection Agency Gene-Tox Program. *Mutat. Res.*, **99**: 303-315.

229 VIOLA, P.L. & CAPUTO, A. (1977) Carcinogenicity studies on vinylidene chloride. *Environ. Health Perspect.*, **21**: 45-47.

230 VOGEL, T.M. & MCCARTY, P.L. (1987) Abiotic and biotic transformations of 1,1,1-trichloroethane under methanogenic conditions. *Environ. Sci. Technol.*, **21**: 1208-1213.

231 WAKEHAM, S.G., GOODWIN, J.T., & DAVIS, A.C. (1983) Distributions and fate of volatile organic compounds in Narragansett Bay, Rhode Island. *Can. J. Fish. Aquat. Sci.*, **40**-(Suppl.2): 304-321.

232 WALKER, W.W., MANNING, C.S., OVERSTREET, R.M., & HAWKINS, W.E. (1985) Development of aquarium fish models for environmental carcinogenesis: an intermittent-flow exposure system for volatile, hydrophobic chemicals. *J. appl. Toxicol.*, **5**: 255-260.

233 WALLACE, L., ZWEIDINGER, R., ERICKSON, M., COOPER, S., WHITAKER, D., & PELLIZZARI, E. (1982) Monitoring individual exposure. Measurements of volatile organic compounds in breathing-zone air, drinking water and exhaled breath. *Environ. Int.*, **8**: 269-282.

234 WALLACE, L., PELLIZZARI, E., HARTWELL, T., ROSENZWEIG, M., ERICKSON, M., SPARACINO, C., & ZELON, H. (1984) Personal exposure to volatile organic compounds. I. Direct measurements in breathing-zone air, drinking water, food, and exhaled breath. *Environ. Res.*, **35**: 293-319.

235 WALLACE, L.A, PELLIZZARI, E., SHELDON, S., HARTWELL, T., SPARACINO, C., & ZELON, H. (1986) The total exposure assessment methodology (TEAM) study: direct measurements of personal exposures through air and water for 600 residents of several US cities. In: Cohen, Y., ed. *Pollutants in a multimedia environment*, New York, London, Plenum Publishing Corporation. pp. 289-315.

236 WANG, T. & LENAHAN, R. (1984) Determination of volatile halocarbons in water by purge-closed loop gas chromatography. *Bull. environ. Contam. Toxicol.*, **32**: 429-438.

237 WANG, T., LENAHAN, R., & KANIK, M. (1985) Impact of trichloroethylene contaminated groundwater discharged to the main canal and Indian river lagoon, Vero Beach, Florida. Bull. environ. Contam. Toxicol., **34**: 578-586.

238 WARNER, C., MODDERMAN, J., FAZIO, T., BEROZA, M., SCHWARTZMAN, G., FOMINAYA, K., & SHERMA, J. (1983) *Food additives analytical manual*, Arlington, Virginia, Association of Official Analytical Chemists, Vol. 1, pp. 348-357.

239 WASKELL, L. (1978) Study of the mutagenicity of anesthetics and their metabolites. Mutat. Res., **57**: 141-153.

240 WAXWEILER, R.J., SMITH, A.H., FALK, H., & TYROLER, H.A. (1981) Excess lung cancer risk in a synthetic chemicals plant. Environ. Health Perspect., **41**: 159-165.

241 WEAST, R.C., ed. (1984) *CRC Handbook of chemistry and physics*, 65th ed., Boca Raton, Florida, CRC Press, p. C-295.

242 WEGMAN, R.C.C., BANK, C.A., & GREVE, P.A. (1981) Environmental pollution by a chemical waste dump. Stud. environ. Sci.,**17**: 349- 357.

243 WESSLING, R.A. & EDWARDS, F.G. (1971) Vinylidene chloride polymers. In: Bikales, N.M., ed. *Encyclopedia of polymer science and technology*, New York, Wiley Interscience, Vol. 14, pp. 540-579.

244 WHO (1984) *Guidelines for drinking-water quality*, Vol. 1 and 2, Geneva, World Health Organization.

245 WOLFF, T., DISTLERATH, L.M., WORTHINGTON, M.T., GROOPMAN, J.D., HAMMONS, G.J., KADLUBAR, F.F., PROUGH, R.A., MARTIN, M.V., & GUENGERICH, F.P. (1985) Substrate specificity of human liver cytochrome P-450 debrisoquine 4-hydroxylase probed using immunochemical inhibition and chemical modeling. Cancer Res., **45**: 2116-2122.

246 YOUNG, D.R., GOSSETT, R.W., BAIRD, R.B., BROWN, D.A., TAYLOR, P.A., & MIILLE, M.J. (1981) Wastewater inputs and marine bioaccumulation of priority pollutant organics off Southern California; In: Jolley, R.L., Brungs, W.A., Cotrivo, J.A. Cumming, R.B., Mattice, J.S., & Jacobs, V.A., ed. *Proceedings of the Fourth Conference on Water Chlorination (Environmental Impact and Health Effects), Pacific Grove, California, 18-23 October, 1981*, Ann Arbor, Michigan, Ann Arbor Science Publishers, Chapter 60, pp. 871-884.

247 ZELLER, H. & PEH, J. (1975) [*Report on the tests of vinylidene chloride for mutagenic effects in Chinese Hamsters after single oral application (chromosomal study)*], Ludwigshafen, BASF Aktiengesellschaft, 12 pp (in German).

248 ZELLER, H., KLIMISCH, J.H., & FREISBERG, K.O. (1979a) [*Report on the determination of acute toxicity (LC_{50}) by inhalation of vinylidene chloride in vapour form in Sprague-Dawley rats (fasting) during a 4-hour exposure period*], Ludwigshafen, BASF Aktiengesellschaft, 14 pp (in German).

References

249 ZELLER, H., KLIMISCH, J.H., & FREISBERG, K.O. (1979b) [*Report on the determination of acute toxicity (LC_{50}) of vinylidene chloride in Sprague-Dawley rats (fed) during a 4-hour exposure*] Ludwigshafen, BASF Aktiengesellschaft, 14 pp. (in German).

250 ZELLER, H., KLIMISCH, J.H., & FREISBERG, K.O. (1979c) [*Report on the determination of acute toxicity (LC_{50}) by inhalation of vinylidene chloride in NMRI mice (fasting) during a 4-hour exposure*] Ludwigshafen, BASF Aktiengesellschaft, 12 pp. (in German).

251 ZELLER, H., KLIMISCH, J.H., & FREISBERG, K.O. (1979d) [*Report on the determination of acute toxicity (LC_{50}) by inhalation of vinylidene chloride in NMRI mice (fed) during a 4-hour exposure*] Ludwigshafen, BASF Aktiengesellschaft, 12 pp. (in German).

RESUME ET CONCLUSIONS, EVALUATION ET RECOMMANDATIONS

1. Résumé et conclusions

1.1 Propriétés, usages et méthodes d'analyse

Le chlorure de vinylidène ($C_2H_2Cl_2$) est un liquide volatil et incolore d'odeur douceâtre. On le stabilise au moyen de *p*-méthoxyphénol afin d'éviter la formation de peroxydes explosifs. Le chlorure de vinylidène est utilisé pour la production de trichloro-1,1,1-éthane, de fibres et de copolymères modacryliques (avec du chlorure de vinyle ou de l'acrylonitrile). On a mis au point des méthodes de chromatographie en phase gazeuse pour la recherche et le dosage du chlorure de vinylidène dans l'air, l'eau ou les emballages, les tissus de l'organisme, les denrées alimentaires et le sol. Le détecteur le plus sensible est le détecteur à capture d'électrons.

1.2 Sources et niveaux d'exposition

Chaque année on libère dans l'atmosphère une quantité de chlorure de vinylidène qui correspond à une proportion allant jusqu'à 5 % de la production totale (soit environ 23 000 tonnes au maximum). La forte tension de vapeur et la faible solubilité dans l'eau de ce produit font qu'il est relativement abondant dans l'atmosphère par rapport aux autres compartiments du milieu. On pense que le chlorure de vinylidène présent dans l'atmosphère a une demi-vie d'environ deux jours.

Dans l'eau, les concentrations sont très faibles. Même dans les eaux résiduaires industrielles, les concentrations sont de l'ordre du µg/litre, c'est-à-dire bien inférieures aux concentrations toxiques pour la faune aquatique, concentrations qui sont de l'ordre du mg/litre. Dans l'eau de boisson non traitée, les concentrations ne sont généralement pas décelables. Dans l'eau potable traitée, la teneur en chlorure de vinylidène est généralement inférieure à 1 µg/litre encore qu'on ait trouvé des échantillons qui en contenaient 20 ≤ g/litre. Dans les denrées alimentaires, les concentrations ne sont généralement pas décelables, le maximum observé étant de 10 µg/kg.

L'exposition professionnelle au chlorure de vinylidène peut se produire soit par inhalation, soit par contamination de la peau ou des yeux. Selon les pays, la dose maximale recommandée ou l'exposition moyenne pondérée en fonction du temps (TWA) se situent dans les limites de 8 à 500 mg/m^3; quelquefois, la dose maximale correspond à la concentration la plus faible qui soit décelable de façon certaine. Les limites d'exposition à court terme vont de 16 à 80 mg/m^3 et les valeurs plafond de 500 à 700 mg/m^3.

1.3 Absorption, distribution, métabolisme et excrétion

Le chlorure de vinylidène peut être absorbé facilement par les voies respiratoires ou digestives chez les mammifères; en revanche on ne dispose pas de renseignements sur l'absorption percutanée. Administré à des rongeurs, le chlorure de vinylidène se répartit largement dans l'organisme de l'animal, les concentrations étant maximales dans le foie et les reins. L'élimination par la voie pulmonaire du chlorure de vinylidène inchangé s'effectue selon un processus au moins biphasé qui dépend de la dose; elle est plus importante aux doses qui provoquent une saturation du métabolisme (c'est-à-dire 600 mg/m^3 environ (150 ppm) chez le rat). Des rats à qui l'on avait administré une dose de chlorure de vinylidène par voie orale et que l'on avait ensuite fait jeûner ont exhalé davantage de cette substance.

Les principales voies du métabolisme ont été identifiées chez le rat. Dans la voie prédominante (phase I), intervient le cytochrome P-450 et il y a formation (vraisemblablement, mais pas forcément par l'intermédiaire d'un époxyde), d'acide monochloracétique. Le chlorure de vinylidène peut stimuler l'activité du cytochrome P-450. Un certain nombre de métabolites de la Phase I peuvent se conjuguer au glutathion ou à la phosphatidyl-éthanolamine avant de subir d'autres transformations. Le métabolisme est plus rapide chez la souris que chez le rat, avec un profil analogue où les dérivés conjugués au glutathion sont relativement plus abondants. On a montré que le chlorure de vinylidène était également métabolisé par le cytochrome P-450 des microsomes humains.

Chez les rongeurs, le métabolisme du chlorure de vinylidène conduit à la déplétion du glutathion et à l'inhibition de la glutathion-S-transférase.

1.4 Effets sur les animaux d'expérience et les systèmes cellulaires

1.4.1 Fixation aux tissus par liaison covalente

Le chlorure de vinylidène radio-marqué se fixe aux tissus hépatiques, rénaux et pulmonaires des rongeurs par liaison covalente et c'est ce phénomène qui déclenche le processus toxique. Les liaisons par covalence et par conséquent la toxicité sont accrues par la déplétion en glutathion et se produisent au niveau du foie et du rein à plus faible dose chez la souris que chez le rat. Un certain nombre de métabolites du chlorure de vinylidène se fixent par liaison covalente aux thiols in vitro.

1.4.2 Toxicité aigue

Les estimations de la CL_{50} aiguë du chlorure de vinylidène varient considérablement, mais cette variation ne masque pas le fait que les souris sont beaucoup plus sensibles à cette substance que les rats ou les hamsters. Les valeurs estimatives de la CL_{50} orale à 4-h varient d'environ 8000 à 128 000 mg/m^3 (2000–32 000 ppm) chez le rat, de 450 à 820 mg/m^3 (115–205 ppm) chez la souris et de 6640–11 780 mg/m^3 (1660–2945 ppm) chez le hamster.

Du fait que la relation entre la concentration et la mortalité n'est pas linéaire, les estimations de la CL_{50} peuvent être entachées d'erreurs. Chez toutes les espèces, la CL_{50} a tendance à être plus faible pour les mâles que pour les femelles et le jeûne (qui provoque une déplétion en glutathion) accroît la toxicité dans tous les cas. Après administration par voie orale les valeurs de la DL_{50} s'établissaient approximativement à 1500 et 100 mh/kilo respectivement chez les rats et les souris. Aprés inhalation, la toxicité s'est manifestée par une irritation des muqueuses, une dépression du système nerveux central et une cardiotoxicité progressive (bradycardie sinusale et arrythmies). On a noté des lésions au niveau du foie, des reins et des poumons. Chez les souris, qui sont plus sensibles que les rats à l'hépatotoxicité et à la néphrotoxicité du chlorure de vinylidène, on a constaté qu'une exposition à des concentrations ne dépassant pas 40 mg/m^3 (10 ppm) pendant 6 heures accroissait les lésions rénales et la réplication de l'ADN. Comme dans le cas de l'inhalation, les principaux organes affectés par l'administration de chlorure de vinylidène par voie orale, sont le foie, les reins et les poumons. Le processus toxique au niveau du foie commence par des altérations au niveau des canaux biliaires et se poursuit par l'apparition de signes d'atteinte mitochondriale. Après quoi il y a lésion du réticulum endoplasmique et mort de la cellule. Il ne semble pas que la toxicité du chlorure de vinylidène pour le foie et le rein soit due à la peroxydation des lipides. Il semblerait plutôt que l'augmentation de la concentration intra-cellulaire des ions calcium soit à l'origine de la toxicité de ce produit pour les hépatocytes.

Les effets toxiques du chlorure de vinylidène dépendent, au moins partiellement, de l'activité du cytochrome P-450 (qui peut également intervenir dans le détoxication) et peuvent être exacerbés par une déplétion en glutathion. L'éthanol et la thyroxine peuvent accroître l'hépatotoxicité; en revanche celle-ci est inhibée par le dithiorcarbe et la (+)-catéchine et modulée par l'acétone.

1.4.3 Etudes à court terme

Des lésions hépatiques et rénales accompagnées, dans une moindre proportion, de lésions pulmonaires ont été observées chez des rongeurs exposés par inhalation à du chlorure de vinylidène à raison de 40 à 800 mg/m^3, 4 à 8 heures par jour, pendant 4 jours ou plus par semaine. Les souris se sont révélées plus sensibles que les rats, les cobayes, les lapins, les chiens et les saïmiris alors que chez les souris, la toxicité variait selon la souche utilisée. En général, les souris femelles étaient moins sensibles que mâles. On a observé une hépatotoxicité chez des rats et des souris exposés de façon intermittente à des concentrations de chlorure de vinylidène respectivement > 800 mg/m^3 (> 200 ppm) ou égales à 220 mg/m^3 (55 ppm). Pour induire une hépatotoxicité par exposition continue durant plusieurs jours, il fallait 240 mg/m^3 (60 ppm) pour les rats et 60 mg/m^3 (15 ppm) pour les souris. Ce traitement intermittant ou continu a également provoqué une néphrotoxicité chez les

Résumé et évaluation

souris. Les souris mâles de la race Swiss se sont montrées particulièrement sensibles à la néphrotoxocité induite par le chlorure de vinylidène. Les mâles n'ont pas survécu à une exposition continue de courte durée à 200 mg de chlorure de vinylidène par m^3 (50 ppm). Chez les chiens, les saïmiris et les rats, le seuil d'hépatotoxicité se situait à environ 80 mg/m^3 (20 ppm) administrés de façon continue sur 90 jours. Des études à court terme (d'une durée d'environ 3 mois) au cours desquelles du chlorure de vinylidène a été administré par voie orale à des rats à des doses allant jusqu'à 20 mg/kg par jour et á des chiens à des doses allant jusqu'à 25 mg/kg, n'ont pas révélé de signes de toxicité, si ce n'est quelques lésions hépatiques infimes et réversibles chez les rats.

1.4.4 Etudes à long terme

Des études à long terme comportant l'inhalation intermittente de chlorure de vinylidène ont révélé que la dose de 300 mg/m^3 (75 ppm) ne produisait que des modifications bénignes et réversibles au niveau du foie chez les rats. A 600 mg/m^3 (150 ppm) c'est-à-dire la dose la plus forte qui soit supportable au cours d'une exposition à long terme, on constatait de nettes lésions hépatiques avec nécrose. On a observé une forte mortalité avec des signes de lésion hépatique chez des souris soumises à une dose de 200 mg/m^3 (50 ppm). La néphrotoxicité était évidente chez la souris après un traitement à long terme à la dose de 100 mg/m^3 (25 ppm). L'administration de chlorure de vinylidène par voie orale à des rats pendant un an à des doses quotidiennes allant jusqu'à 300 mg/kg n'a produit que de minimes anomalies hépatiques. Il n'est pas possible de tirer de ces données une valeur précise de la dose sans effet observable. Une autre étude a révélé des signes d'inflammation rénale et de nécrose hépatique chez des rats et des souris soumis à une administration orale prolongée de chlorure de vinylidène à des doses quotidiennes respectives de 5 mg/kg et 2 mg/kg.

1.4.5 Génotoxicité et cancérogénicité

On a constaté que le chlorure de vinylidène était mutagène pour les bactéries et les levures, mais seulement en présence d'un système mammalien d'activation métabolique microsomique (S9). Le composé a provoqué une synthèse anarchique de l'ADN dans des hépatocytes isolés de rats ainsi qu'une augmentation de la fréquence des échanges entre chromatides soeurs et des aberrations chromosomiques dans des cultures cellulaires additionnées de S9. Par contre, on n'a pas observé d'accroissement des mutations géniques chez les mammifères. Il a été fait état d'une augmentation légère mais statistiquement significative de la liaison à l'ADN après exposition in vivo. Cette liaison était plus importante dans les cellules de souris que dans celles de rats et également plus importante dans les reins que dans le foie après une exposition de 6 heures à des concentrations de 40 et 200 mg de chlorure de vinylidène/m^3 (10 et 50 ppm). En outre, le chlorure de vinylidène augmentait légèrement la synthèse anarchique de l'ADN dans le rein de la souris. On a relevé aucun signe de mutation létale dominante ou d'effets cytogénétiques après exposition in vivo de rongeurs, sauf dans le cas d'une étude au cours de laquelle on a observé des aberrations chromosomiques dans la moëlle osseuse de hansters chinois.

Des études de cancérogénicité ont été effectuées sur trois espèces animales (rats, souris et hamsters). Chez des souris mâles de race Swiss, on a relevé un net effet cancérogène (adénocarcinome rénal) après exposition prolongée intermittente à des concentrations de 100 ou de 200 mg/m^3 de chlorure de vinylidène (25 ou 50 ppm), mais pas aux concentrations de 0 ou 40 mg/m^3 (0 ou 10 ppm).

Il est possible que ces tumeurs rénales soient liées d'une manière ou d'une autre à la néphrotoxicité observée et que des atteintes rénales répétées puissent conduire directement à une réaction cancérogène selon un mécanisme non génotoxique ou qu'elles facilitent l'expression de l'activité génotoxique de certains métabolites chez cette espèce, pour ce sexe et au niveau de cet organe. Toutefois, cette conclusion reste hypothétique du fait que les données disponibles sur les effets génétiques *in vivo* sont limitées et que le chlorure de vinylidène a pu jouer le rôle d'initiateur.

Dans la même étude, on a constaté une augmentation statistique de l'incidence des tumeurs pulmonaires (principalement des adénomes chez les souris des deux sexes) et des cancers mammaires (chez les femelles) mais on a pas observé de relation entre la dose et la réponse. Chez des rats adultes exposés par inhalation au chlorure de vinylidène, on a signalé une légère augmentation des tumeurs mammaires sans relation avec la dose ainsi qu'une augmentation modérée des leucémies lorsque les rats étaient exposés à la substance in utero puis après leur naissance. Il n'a pas été possible d'évaluer les résultats.

1.4.6 *Toxicité pour la fonction de reproduction*

Aucun effet n'a été observé sur la fécondité de rats exposés en permanence à du chlorure de vinylidène (jusqu'à 200 mg/litre ou 200 ppm) ajouté à leur eau de boisson. Des rats et des souris qui avaient inhalé jusqu'à 1200 mg de chlorure de vinylidène par m^3 (300 ppm) pendant 22 à 23 heures, à différents stades de l'organogenèse, n'ont pas produit de foetus présentant des anomalies autres que celles qui peuvent être attribuées à une action toxique sur la mère.

Des rats et des lapins ont inhalé 7 h/jour 640 mg de chlorure de vinylidène par m^3 (160 ppm) ou absorbé par voie orale environ 40 mg/kilo de cette substance au cours des stades critiques de la gestation sans que les embryons ou les foetus présentent d'anomalies à ces doses, inférieures aux doses toxiques pour la mère. Toutefois, des anomalies ont été constatées sur les embryons et les foetus aux doses toxiques pour la mère, comme l'a montré la réduction du gain de poids.

1.5 *Effets sur l'homme*

Des concentrations de chlorure de vinylidène de l'ordre de 16 000 mg/m^3 (4000 ppm) provoquent une intoxication pouvant entraîner une perte de connaissance. Additionné de stabilisateur, le chlorure de vinylidène est également irritant pour les voies respiratoires, les yeux et la peau. A la suite d'expositions prolongées ou répétées à des doses infra-anesthésiques, on a signalé l'apparition de lésions rénales et hépatiques. Il est difficile d'évaluer les résultats obtenus par les études épidémiologiques en raison de l'effectif limité des cohortes, d'une exposition simultanée au chlorure de vinyle et du fait qu'on n'a pas suffisamment tenu compte du tabagisme. On n'a pas constaté d'augmentation statistiquement significative dans l'incidence des cancers chez les personnes exposées au chlorure de vinylidène, mais il est vrai que les études épidémiologiques présentaient des insuffisances; aussi n'est-il pas possible d'en conclure qu'il n'existe aucun risque de cancérogénicité. On ne dispose d'aucun renseignement concernant les effets du chlorure de vinylidène sur la fonction de reproduction humaine.

2. Evaluation des effets sur l'environnement et des risques pour la santé humaine

2.1 Evaluation des effets sur l'environnement

Par suite de la volatilité du chlorure de vinylidène, c'est l'atmosphère qui est le compartiment du milieu où il est le plus abondant. La demi-vie du chlorure de vinylidène dans la troposphère est vraisemblablement d'environ deux jours, aussi ce composé ne contribue-t-il probablement pas à la réduction de la couche d'ozone stratosphérique. Lessivage et volatilisation font du sol et des sédiments des compartiments où le chlorure de vinylidène n'est présent qu'en petites quantités et cet hydrocarbure chloré n'apparaît qu'en quantité minime dans le milieu aquatique du fait de sa volatilisation rapide. On ignore si la dégradation de composés tel que le trichloréthylène et le perchloréthylène, souvent présents dans l'eau, contribuent de manière notable à la concentration du chlorure de vinylidène dans l'environnement.

La concentration du chlorure de vinylidène dans l'environnement et les valeurs de la toxicité aiguë pour les poissons et la daphnie montrent que les risques d'intoxication aiguë sont minimes pour la faune aquatique. On ne dispose pas de données suffisantes sur la toxicité à long terme pour évaluer les effets sublétaux sur les organismes aquatiques qui vivent à proximité de sources relativement importantes de contamination par le chlorure de vinylidène, qu'il s'agisse d'eaux souterraines contaminées ou d'eaux résiduaires municipales ou industrielles.

2.1 Évaluation des risques pour la santé humaine

2.1.1 Niveau d'exposition

La population générale n'est exposée qu'à de très faibles teneurs de chlorure de vinylidène. La concentration maximale qui ait été signalée dans l'eau de boisson est de 20 µg par litre, encore que l'exposition individuelle moyenne pour les citoyens des Etats-Unis d'Amérique par l'intermédiaire de l'eau de boisson soit estimée à moins de 0,01 µg par jour. Il n'y a pas de chlorure de vinylidène en concentrations décelables dans les denrées alimentaires et en tout état de cause on n'a pas signalé de teneurs supérieures à 10 µg/kg. On ignore quelles sont les concentrations dans les denrées alimentaires constituées d'organismes aquatiques mais elles sont vraisemblablement insignifiantes (section 10.1). Dans l'air ambiant on a signalé des concentrations en chlorure de vinylidène allant jusqu'à 52 µg/m^3 (dans le périmètre d'une zone industrielle). Des concentrations médianes dans l'air urbain de 20 ng/m^3 et de 8,7 µg/m^3 ont été signalées aux Etats-Unis, respectivement dans des zones non industrielles et dans des zones industrielles.

L'exposition professionnelle se produit notamment lors de la production et de la polymérisation du chlorure de vinylidène. C'est principalement par la voie respiratoire que cette substance pénètre dans l'organisme et les limites maximales recommandées ou réglementées pendant une journée de travail vont de 8 à 500 mg/m^3 (ou la concentration la plus faible qui soit décelable par une méthode fiable), selon les pays. Les limites d'exposition à court terme vont de 16 à 80 mg/m^3 et les valeurs plafonds de 50 à 700 mg/m^3. La concentration atmosphérique de chlorure de vinylidène en atmosphère confinée à laquelle certains travailleurs peuvent être exposés, ne dépasse pas 8 mg/m^3.

2.2 Effets aigus

Chez l'homme, l'inhalation de fortes concentrations de chlorure de vinylidène (très approximativement, supérieures ou égales au seuil olfactif maximal de 4000 mg/m^3) peuvent vraisemblablement provoquer une dépression du système nerveux central susceptible d'évoluer vers le coma. En se basant sur la toxicité aiguë de ce composé chez l'animal, on pense que les effets toxiques du chlorure de vinylidène peuvent se manifester au niveau du foie, des reins ou des poumons bien en dessous du seuil olfactif minimum qui se situe aux environs de 2000 mg/m^3. L'exposition au chlorure de vinylidène peut provoquer une irritation des yeux, des voies respiratoires supérieures (à la concentration de 100 mg/m^3 chez l'homme), et de la peau, encore que cet effet irritant soit, semble-t-il, dû en partie au para-méthoxyphénol utilisé comme stabilisateur.

Chez la souris, qui est plus sensible que le rat aux effets hépatotoxiques et néphrotoxiques du chlorure de vinylidène, on a constaté une atteinte rénale après exposition à des concentrations ne dépassant pas 40 mg de chlorure de vinylidène par m^3 (soit 10 ppm) pendant 6 heures. On a également observé une hépato-toxicité et une néphrotoxicité notables chez le rat. Lorsque les animaux sont à jeun, ce qui a pour effet d'exacerber la toxicité, l'exposition au chlorure de vinylidène à des teneurs de 600 mg/m^3 (150 ppm) et de 800 mg/m^3 (200 ppm) pendant 6 heures a provoqué chez le rat des effets toxiques, respectivement au niveau du foie et du rein. Des études sur le rat ont montré que l'ingestion d'alcool avant l'exposition peut stimuler le métabolisme et exacerber la toxicité du chlorure de vinylidène. La toxicité agiuë dépend de l'espèce, du sexe, de la souche et de l'état alimentaire de l'animal. Chez le rat et la souris, les différences de sensibilité interspécifiques sont liées à l'activité du métabolisme oxydatif. S'il n'est pas possible de déterminer qui du rat ou de la souris constitue le meilleur modèle pour l'être humain, toujours est-il que le métabolisme des micro-somes hépatiques est, chez l'homme, quantitativement analogue à celui du rat, espèce relativement peu sensible aux effets du chlorure de vinylidène. Rien n'indique qu'il existe une différence de nature entre l'homme et les rongeurs pour ce qui est du métabolisme oxidatif du chlorure de vinylidène.

Il semblerait que la marge entre la concentration toxique chez l'animal (40 mg/m^3 pour la souris) et les limites d'exposition professionnelle fixées par certains pays puisse être insuffisante, voire nulle.

2.3 Effets à long terme et génotoxicité

Une exposition prolongée ou des expositions de courte durée répétées à des doses infra-anesthésiques peuvent provoquer des lésions rénales ou hépatiques. Sur la base d'études à long terme chez l'animal, dans des conditions reproduisant une exposition professionnelle, on a observé chez le rat, des altérations au niveau du foie à une dose de 300 mg/m^3 (75 ppm). Chez la souris, des lésions rénales et hépatiques ont été observées respectivement à 100 mg/m^3 (25 ppm) et 200 mg/m^3 (50 ppm). La sensibilité aux effets toxiques observée au cours des différentes études présente des variations considérables.

Le chlorure de vinylidène n'affecte pas, semble-t-il, la capacité de reproduction chez l'animal et ne semble pas non plus comporter de risques d'embryotoxicité ou de tératogénicité aux doses inférieures à celles qui seraient toxiques pour la mère, mais on n'a pas effectué d'études de ce type chez l'homme. Aux doses toxiques pour la mère – à en juger par une réduction du gain de poids – on a observé des effets toxiques sur l'embryon et le foetus et des anomalies foetales.

Le chlorure de vinylidène est mutagène pour les bactéries et les levures en présence d'un système métabolique de mammifère. Certaines cellules mammaliennes se révèlent également sensibles *in vitro* aux effets mutagènes et aux lésions de l'ADN. La plupart des études *in vivo* effectuées sur des rats n'ont pas permis d'observer d'effets génotoxiques manifestes, à en juger par les tests de létalité dominante et certains critères cytogénétiques mais on a tout de même signalé la présence d'aberrations chromosomiques dans les cellules de la moelle osseuse de hamsters chinois. La liaison à l'ADN et sa réparation sont décelables *in vivo* chez les rongeurs mais en proportion minime. Les études génétiques *in vivo* incitent donc à penser qu'il existe une certaine toxicité génique mais, dans la majorité des cas, il s'agit d'effets non décelables ou minimes.

Plusieurs épreuves de cancérogénicité ont été effectuées sur trois espèces d'animaux d'expérience (souris, rats et hamsters) selon différentes voies d'administration. Malheureusement, la plupart de ces études laissent beaucoup à désirer tant au niveau de leur conception que de l'évaluation du risque cancérogène. Aucun effet cancérogène significatif n'a été observé chez des rats qui recevaient ce composé par la voie orale. Chez des rats adultes exposés par inhalation, on a signalé une augmentation de la fréquence des tumeurs mammaires qui n'était toutefois pas liée à la dose. Une légère augmentation de la fréquence des leucémies a été également observée, lorsque les rats étaient exposés in utero ou après leur naissance. Ces observations n'ont pas pu être évaluées. Lors d'une étude sur la souris, on a observé chez les mâles une augmentation de l'incidence des adénocarcinome du rein aux doses de 200 et 100 mg/m^3 (50 et 25 ppm), mais aucun effet de ce genre aux doses de 40 et 0 mg/m^3 (10 et 0 ppm). Au cours de la même étude, une augmentation statistiquement significative de l'incidence des tumeurs pulmonaires (essentiellement des adénomes chez les deux sexes) et des carcinomes mammaires (chez les femelles) a été observée, sans toutefois qu'il y ait de relation dose-réponse.

Il est possible que ces tumeurs rénales soient liées d'une manière ou d'une autre à la néphrotoxicité observée et que des atteintes rénales répétées puissent conduire directement à une réaction cancérogène selon un mécanisme non-génotoxique ou qu'elle facilite l'expression de l'activité génotoxique de certains métabolites chez cette espèce, pour ce sexe et au niveau de cet organe. Toutefois, cette conclusion reste hypothétique du fait que l'on ne possède pas suffisamment de résultats sur la relation dose-réponse pour ce qui est des effets génétiques *in vivo;* en outre, le chlorure de vinylidène a pu jouer le rôle d'initiateur lors d'un test cutané en deux phases sur la souris.

Les études épidémiologiques ne fournissent pas de résultats statistiquement significatifs qui puissent permettre de conclure à un accroissement du risque de cancer à la suite d'une exposition professionnelle au chlorure de vinylidène, toutefois ces études présentent des insuffisances telles qu'on ne peut procéder à une évaluation convenable du risque de cancérogénicité pour l'homme.

Même si les estimations effectuées par divers auteurs écartent l'idée d'une surmortalité par cancer en arguant qu'il s'agit d'une pure coincidence(en raison du petit nombre de cas et du faible effectif des cohortes), il n'est pas inutile de préciser que les résultats obtenus sont systématiquement supérieurs aux prévisions. Ainsi, dans les deux études de cohorte dont il est fait état, on a observé

Résumé et évaluation

un cancer du poumon dans 7 cas, alors qu'on aurait dû avoir 3,16 décès. On ne peut pas écarter ce résultat, mais il ne faut pas oublier l'existence, dans une étude, d'une exposition concomitante au chlorure de vinylidène. Etant donné que les cohortes ont été constituées sur la base d'une exposition au chlorure de vinylidène, on peut se trouver dans l'impossibilité d'éliminer d'autres expositions parasites.

Les données de morbidité indiquées (y compris un cas de cancer du testicule) ne sont pas dénuées d'intérêt. Selon les auteurs, la forte morbidité hépatique serait imputable à la consommation d'alcool. Cette hypothèse ne tient pas, puisque la consommation d'alcool de l'ensemble des personnes étudiées (pas seulement les cas identifiés) n'a pas été évaluée.

3. Recommandations

3.1 Recommandations en vue de travaux futurs

Il faudrait disposer d'une meilleure estimation de la production annuelle mondiale de chlorure de vinylidène ainsi que des quantités de cette substance qui pénètrent dans l'environnement à partir de l'ensemble des sources de pollution, que le composé soit libéré tel quel ou qu'il résulte de la décomposition d'autres produits chimiques.

Les prévisions relatives à sa destiné dans l'environnement reposent sur un nombre limité de données expérimentales. Il faudrait de nouvelles données sur les produits de dégradation et de transformation de ce composé dans l'air, le sol, l'eau et les sédiments ainsi que sur son métabolisme chez des espèces non-mammaliennes représentatives.

Il conviendrait d'effectuer des études de toxicité à long terme chez diverses espèces aquatiques représentatives (poissons, crustacés et mollusques), selon divers critères pathologiques.

Il faut également définir de manière plus précise, afin d'établir des critères de sécurité en matière d'exposition, quels sont, chez l'animal et chez l'homme, les mécanismes des effets toxiques résultant d'une exposition de brève ou prolongée au chlorure de vinylidène.

Il faudrait exploiter de manière plus complète les données existantes sur la cancérogénicité. Si l'on envisage d'autres études de cancérogénicité, elles devront être menées selon un protocole expérimental reconnu, pendant toute l'existence des sujets, ce protocole étant conçu de manière à tenir compte des propriétés particulières du chlorure de vinylidène. Ces études doivent notamment prendre en considération la courte demi-vie du produit dans l'organisme, l'importance de l'âge au début de l'exposition, la durée de l'exposition quotidienne et autres données susceptibles d'aider à la détermination des doses à administrer. Les espèces et les souches d'animaux de laboratoire devront être soigneusement sélectionnées. Il serait également très utile de disposer de données de toxicité ainsi que de données métaboliques et pharmacocinétiques sur ces animaux.

Il faudrait effectuer des études longitudinales à long terme sur la morbidité et la mortalité au sein de populations prises au hasard et qui sont exposées au chlorure de vinylidène.

Des études épidémiologiques sont nécessaires pour permettre l'évaluation des effets de l'exposition au chlorure de vinylidène (notamment une exposition prolongée à de faibles doses) dans les populations humaines. Il est tout particulièrement important de disposer de données sur des effets tels que les affections cérébrovasculaires prématurées et le cancer. En outre, les études qui seront effectuées devront tenir dûment compte de facteurs de confusion tels que le tabagisme et la consommation d'alcool (éventuellement selon un système cas/témoin).

Afin d'apprécier l'effet de l'action réglementaire menée au cours des dernières années, il conviendrait de confronter les résultats des études en cours aux données rétrospectives.

Pour résoudre le problème que posent les faibles effectifs du personnel sur les lieux de production, on pourrait, pour les investigations en cours comme pour les investigations futures, recourir à des études multicentriques avec regroupement des données. Il faudra également étudier sur l'animal d'expérience si la *N*-acétylcystéine, un agent sulfhydrilé présente un intérêt pour le traitement des intoxications par le chlorure de vinylidène.

Il est nécessaire de comparer la pharmacocinétique et le métabolisme du chlorure de vinylidène tant *in vivo* qu'*in vitro* spécialement au niveau du rein, du foie et des poumons chez diverses espèces d'animaux d'expérience et chez l'homme, afin de pouvoir mieux interpréter les résultats fournis par les études de toxicité in vivo. Il faut également obtenir des données sur la génotoxicité potentielle du chlorure de vinylidène au site de la cancérogénèse, parallèlement sur plusieurs espèces, afin de voir si un mécanisme génétique est en cause.

Compte tenu des observations neurotoxicologiques dont il est fait état dans la présente analyse, il paraît nécessaire d'étudier le rôle des systèmes de modulation dans la pathogénèse de l'intoxication par le chlorure de vinylidène.

3.2 Protection personnelle et traitement des intoxications

3.2.1 Protection personnelle

Dans l'industrie, où peuvent se produire des expositions de brèves durées par inhalation au dessus des limites recommandées, il conviendrait d'utiliser des masques faciaux avec cartouche filtrante pour se protéger des vapeurs organiques et, si nécessaire en cas d'urgence, des masques respiratoires avec arrivée d'air. Les personnes qui manipulent du chlorure de vinylidène devront porter des vêtements protecteurs ainsi que des lunettes spéciales; cet équipement devra être correctement entretenu afin de protéger le corps contre tout contact. Dans les ateliers, on assurera une ventilation permanente et l'on disposera des grilles d'aération munies de filtres là où des déversements accidentels ou des fuites risquent de se produire. Il est recommandé de surveiller les émissions de chlorure de vinylidène au cours des opérations de remplissage. En cas de fuite, on procédera à l'évaporation directe du produit s'il s'agit d'une fuite mineure ou à son évaporation contrôlée en présence d'une mousse synthétique s'il s'agit d'une fuite plus importante. On pourra disperser la vapeur de chlorure de vinylidène à partir de cette mousse par pulvérisation d'eau.

3.2.2 Traitement des intoxications humaines

En cas d'exposition excessive ou d'ingestion, il faut s'adresser à un médecin. Il faut veiller particulièrement aux poumons, à la peau et aux yeux du fait des propriétés irritantes du chlorure de vinylidène. Il importe de surveiller les fonctions cardiaque, hépatique et rénale ainsi que le système nerveux central. Les données obtenues sur l'animal d'expérience montrent que le chlorure de vinylidène accroît notablement la sensibilité aux arythmies cardiaques induites par l'adrénaline, de sorte que ce produit est à éviter. En cas d'hypotension grave, on pourra procéder à une transfusion de sang total ou d'un succédané du plasma. Il n'existe aucun antidote.

En cas d'intoxication par inhalation de chlorure de vinylidène, il faut maintenir le malade à l'air libre en semi-décubitus ventral. On dégagera les voies aériennes et l'on placera le malade sous oxygène en cas de stupeur ou de coma. Si nécessaire, on procédera à la respiration artificielle.

En cas d'ingestion de chlorure de vinylidène, rincer la bouche avec de l'eau. Ne pas faire vomir le malade car il y a risque d'aspiration du chlorure de vinylidène dans le larynx et les poumons. Un lavage d'estomac ou l'administration par voie orale de charbon actif ou de paraffine liquide peut contribuer à réduire la biodisponibilité du chlorure de vinylidène si on procède à ce traitement dans l'heure qui suit l'ingestion, l'effet bénéfique étant encore sensible après 4 heures.

Si les yeux ont été atteints par du chlorure de vinylidène, les rincer immédiatement à l'eau pendant plus de 15 minutes et consulter un médecin.

En cas d'exposition cutanée, ôter les vêtements souillés et laver la peau à l'eau et au savon.

RESUMEN Y CONCLUSIONES, EVALUACION Y RECOMENDACIONES

1. Resumen y conclusiones

1.1. Propiedades, usos y métodos analíticos

El cloruro de vinilideno ($C_2H_2Cl_2$) es un líquido volátil e incoloro con un olor dulzón. Se estabiliza con p-metoxifenol para impedir la formación de peróxidos explosivos. El cloruro de vinilideno se usa para producir 1,1,1-tricloroetano y para formar fibras modacrílicas y copolímeros (con cloruro de vinilo o acrilonitrilo). Se han puesto a punto métodos de cromatografía de gases para analizar el cloruro de vinilideno en el aire, el agua, las películas para envoltorios, los tejidos orgánicos, los alimentos y el suelo. El método más sensible de detección es la captura electrónica.

1.2. Fuentes y niveles de exposición

Todos los años ingresa en la atmósfera alrededor del 5% del cloruro de vinilideno producido (que representa un máximo cercano a 23 000 toneladas). La elevada presión de vapor y la baja solubilidad en agua favorecen concentraciones atmosféricas relativamente elevadas en comparación con otros "compartimentos" ambientales. Se cree que el cloruro de vinilideno tiene una semivida en la atmósfera de aproximadamente dos días.

Los niveles ambientales en el agua son sumamente bajos. Incluso en aguas residuales industriales sin tratar, las concentraciones pasan raras veces del orden de los µg/litro, lo que está muy por debajo del margen de mg/litro de toxicidad para los organismos acuáticos. Los niveles en el agua de bebida sin tratar no suelen ser detectables. En las aguas potables tratadas, se ha encontrado que el nivel de cloruro de vinilideno suele ser < de 1 µg/litro, si bien se han encontrado muestras que contienen hasta 20 µg/litro. Los niveles de cloruro de vinilideno en los alimentos normalmente no son detectables, siendo la concentración máxima observada de 10 μg/kg.

La exposición profesional al cloruro de vinilideno se da principalmente por inhalación, aunque también puede producirse contaminación por la piel o los ojos. Según los países, el límite de exposición máximo recomendado o promedio ponderado en función del tiempo se encuentra entre 8 y 500 mg/m^3, o es la concentración más baja detectable con cierto margen de confianza. Los límites de exposición a corto plazo varían entre 16 y 80 mg/m^3 y los valores máximos varían entre 50 y 700 mg/m^3.

1.3. Absorción, distribución, metabolismo y excreción

El cloruro de vinilideno puede absorberse rápidamente por la vía respiratoria y oral en mamíferos; no se dispone de datos sobre la absorción cutánea. El cloruro de vinilideno se distribuye por todo el organismo del roedor y alcanza concentraciones máximas en el hígado y el riñón. La eliminación pulmonar de cloruro de vinilideno sin modificar es cuando menos bifásica y dependiente de la dosis, siendo de mayor importancia en el caso de dosis que saturan el metabolismo (> unos 600 mg/m^3 (< 150 ppm) por inhalación en la rata). En la rata sometida a ayuno se observó una reducción en el metabolismo de la dosis oral y un nivel consiguiente mayor de cloruro de vinilideno exhalado.

Se han caracterizado las principales vías metabólicas en la rata. El metabolismo predominante de la fase I entraña la participación del citocromo P-450 y la formación (posible pero no necesariamente por medio de un epóxido) de ácido monocloroacético. El cloruro de vinilideno puede inducir actividad de citocromo P-450. Varios metabolitos de la fase I se conjugan con glutatión y/o con fosfatidil etanolamina antes de sufrir ulteriores modificaciones. El metabolismo es más rápido en el ratón que en la rata, lo que origina un perfil metabólico semejante con una proporción relativamente mayor de derivados del glutatión por conjugación. Se ha demostrado que el citocromo P-450 de microsomas humanos también metaboliza el cloruro de vinilideno.

Resumen y evaluación

El metabolismo del cloruro de vinilideno en roedores lleva al agotamiento de las reservas de glutatión y a la inhibición de la actividad de la glutatión-S-transferasa.

1.4. Efectos en animales de experimentación y sistemas celulares

1.4.1 Enlaces covalentes en tejidos

Los marcadores radiactivos derivados del [^{14}C]-cloruro de vinilideno forman enlaces covalentes en el hígado, el riñón y el pulmón de los roedores, lo que va asociado a toxicidad en esos órganos. El enlace covalente y la toxicidad se agravan con el agotamiento del glutatión y se producen en el hígado y el riñón a dosis inferiores en ratones que en ratas. Se ha observado in vitro que varios metabolitos del cloruro de vinilideno establecen enlaces covalentes con tioles.

1.4.2 Toxicidad aguda

Aunque las estimaciones de la CL$_{50}$ aguda para el cloruro de vinilideno varían considerablemente, esta variación no enmascara el hecho de que el ratón es mucho más sensible a la sustancia que la rata o el criceto. Los valores estimados de la CL$_{50}$ a las 4 h variaron desde aproximadamente 8000 hasta 128 000 mg/m^3 (2000–32 000 ppm) en ratas alimentadas, 460–820 mg/m^3 (115–205 ppm) en ratones alimentados y 6640–11 780 mg/m^3 (1660–2945 ppm) en cricetos alimentados. Pueden existir imprecisiones en los cálculos de la CL$_{50}$ debido a que la relación concentración-mortalidad no es de carácter lineal. En todas las especies, los machos parecían tener valores de CL$_{50}$ más bajos que las hembras, y el ayuno (que agota las reservas de glutatión) aumentó la toxicidad en las tres especies. Tras la administración oral, los valores de la DL$_{50}$ fueron aproximadamente 1500 y 200 mg/kg en ratas y ratones alimentados, respectivamente. La toxicidad aguda por inhalación en animales de laboratorio se manifestó en forma de irritación de las mucosas, depresión del sistema nervioso central y cardiotoxicidad progresiva (bradicardia sinusal y arritmias). Se observaron lesiones en el hígado, el riñón y el pulmón. En el ratón, que es más sensible que la rata a la toxicidad hepática y renal del cloruro de vinilideno, la exposición a dosis tan reducidas como 40 mg de cloruro de vinilideno/m^3 (10 ppm) durante 6 h indujo lesiones renales y aumento de la replicación del ADN. Como en el caso de la inhalación, los principales órganos afectados por la ingestión de cloruro de vinilideno son el hígado, el riñón y el pulmón. La cadena de procesos que llevan a la hepatotoxicidad parece comenzar por un cambio temprano en los canalículos biliares, que se ve seguido por síntomas de lesiones mitocondriales. A continuación se producen lesiones en el retículo endoplasmático y la muerte celular. La toxicidad hepática y renal inducida por el cloruro de vinilideno no parece estar causada por peroxidación lipídica. El aumento de las concentraciones intracelulares de Ca^{++} puede ser en parte responsable de la toxicidad para el hepatocito.

Los efectos tóxicos del cloruro de vinilideno dependen, al menos parcialmente, de la actividad del citocromo P-450 (que también puede participar en la detoxificación) y pueden agravarse por el agotamiento de las reservas de glutatión. La hepatotoxicidad puede ser intensificada por el etanol y la tiroxina, inhibida por el ditiocarbo y la (+)-catequina y modulada por la acetona.

1.3 Estudios a corto plazo

En estudios a corto plazo se han observado lesiones hepáticas, renales y, en menor grado, pulmonares en roedores expuestos por inhalación al cloruro de vinilideno a una concentración de 40–800 mg/m^3 durante 4–8 h/día, 4 o más días/semana. El ratón demostró ser más sensible que la rata, el cobayo, el conejo, el perro y el mono ardilla, y la toxicidad fue distinta de unas familias de ratones a otras. En general, las hembras eran menos sensibles que los machos. Se ha comunicado la aparición de hepatotoxicidad en la rata y el ratón expuestos intermitentemente a concentraciones de cloruro de vinilideno > 800 mg/m^3 (> 200 ppm) y 220 mg/m^3 (55 ppm), respectivamente. Los niveles necesarios para producir hepatotoxicidad por exposición continua durante varios días fueron 240 mg/m^3 (60 ppm) para la rata y 60 mg/m^3 (15 ppm) para el ratón. Estos tratamientos intermitentes y continuos también provocaron nefrotoxicidad en el ratón. El ratón suizo macho resultó ser especialmente propenso a la toxicidad renal inducida por cloruro de vinilideno. El ratón macho no sobrevivió a una exposición continua a corto plazo a 200 mg de cloruro de vinilideno/m^3 (50 ppm). El nivel aparente de no observación de efectos de hepatotoxicidad en el perro, el mono ardilla y la rata fue de aproximadamente 80 mg/m^3 (20 ppm) administrados en exposición continua durante 90 días. En estudios de dosificación oral a corto plazo (aproximadamente 3 meses) en la rata (hasta 20 mg/kg diarios) y el perro (hasta 25 mg/kg diarios) no se observó prueba alguna de toxicidad aparte de una mínima lesión hepática reversible en la rata.

1.4.4 Estudios a largo plazo

Los estudios a largo plazo de exposición intermitente al cloruro de vinilideno por inhalación revelaron que 300 mg/m^3 (75 ppm) sólo causaban ligeras lesiones hepáticas reversibles en la rata. A 600 mg/m^3 (150 ppm), la dosis más alta de exposición a largo plazo que puede tolerar la rata, se apreció lesión hepática con necrosis. En el ratón se observó una elevada tasa de mortalidad con signos de lesión hepática a 200 mg/m^3 (50 ppm). Se observó toxicidad para el riñón en el tratamiento a largo plazo de ratones con 100 mg/m^3 (25 ppm). La administración de hasta 30 mg/kg al día de cloruro de vinilideno a la rata durante un año volvió a producir cambios hepáticos mínimos. A partir de estos datos no se puede determinar claramente el nivel de no observación de efectos. En otro estudio se observaron ciertas pruebas de que podía inducirse inflamación renal y necrosis hepática en la rata y el ratón, respectivamente, tras la administración oral a largo plazo de cloruro de vinilideno a dosis diarias de 5 mg/kg y 2 mg/kg, respectivamente.

1.4.5 Genotoxicidad y carcinogenicidad

Se observó que el cloruro de vinilideno es mutagénico para bacterias y levaduras sólo en presencia de un sistema de activación metabólica de microsomas de mamíferos (S9). El compuesto indujo síntesis no programada de ADN en hepatocitos aislados de rata y aumentó la frecuencia de intercambio de cromátidas hermanas y de aberraciones cromosómicas en cultivos celulares con S9. En cambio, no se observó aumento en la mutación de genes de mamíferos. Se ha comunicado un aumento pequeño pero estadísticamente significativo del enlace al ADN después de la exposición *in vivo*. El enlace al ADN fue más frecuente en células de ratón que de rata y mayor en el riñón que en el hígado tras exposiciones de 6 h a 40 y 200 mg de cloruro de vinilideno/m^3 (10 y 50 ppm). Además, el cloruro de vinilideno aumentaba ligeramente la síntesis no programada de ADN en el riñón de ratón. No se observó prueba alguna de efectos letales dominantes o de efectos citogenéticos tras la exposición *in vivo* de roedores a excepción de un estudio que demuestra la inducción de aberraciones cromosómicas en la médula ósea del criceto chino.

Se han llevado a cabo estudios de carcinogenicidad en tres especies animales (rata, ratón y criceto). En el ratón suizo macho, se vieron signos claros de carcinogenicidad (adenocarcinoma del riñón) tras una exposición intermitente a largo plazo a 100 ó 200 mg de cloruro de vinilideno/m^3 (25 ó 50 ppm) pero no a 0 ó 40 mg/m^3 (0 ó 10 ppm).

Los tumores de riñón pueden guardar alguna relación con la citotoxicidad renal observada y es posible que la lesión renal repetida lleve directamente a la respuesta carcinogénica por un mecanismo no genotóxico o bien que facilite la expresión del potencial genotóxico de los metabolitos en esta especie, sexo y órgano en concreto. No obstante, esta conclusión es dudosa a la luz de los escasos datos disponibles sobre los efectos genéticos *in vivo* y el descubrimiento de que el cloruro de vinilideno podía haber actuado como iniciador.

En el mismo estudio, se observaron incidencias estadísticamente mayores de tumor del pulmón (principalmente adenomas en el ratón de ambos sexos) y carcinomas mamarios (en hembras), pero no se encontraron relaciones dosis-respuesta. En rata adulta expuesta por inhalación, se comunicó un ligero aumento independiente de la dosis de tumores de la mama, así como un pequeño aumento de la leucemia cuando se exponía a la rata *in utero* y recién nacida. Estas observaciones no pudieron evaluarse.

1.4.6 *Efectos sobre la reproducción*

No se encontró efecto alguno sobre la fecundidad de la rata continuamente expuesta al cloruro de vinilideno (hasta 200 mg/litro, 200 ppm) en el agua de bebida. La inhalación de hasta 1200 mg de cloruro de vinilideno/m^3 (300 ppm), durante 22-23 horas, por la

Resumen y evaluación

rata y el ratón durante diversos periodos de la organogénesis no indujo anomalías fetales que no pudieran atribuirse a la toxicidad materna.

La inhalación de hasta 640 mg de cloruro de vinilideno/m^3 (160 ppm) durante 7 h/día en ratas y conejos o la ingestión de aproximadamente 40 mg/kg al día en la rata durante periodos críticos de la gestación no ejercieron efecto alguno sobre los embriones o los fetos en niveles inferiores al que produce la toxicidad materna, pero se observaron toxicidad embrionaria y fetal y anomalías fetales cuando se alcanzó el nivel que produce toxicidad en la madre, como lo demostró la menor velocidad de aumento de peso.

1.5. Efectos en el hombre

Una concentración de cloruro de vinilideno de 16 000 mg/m^3 (4000 ppm) provoca una intoxicación que puede llevar a la pérdida del conocimiento. El cloruro de vinilideno estabilizado es también irritante para el tracto respiratorio, los ojos y la piel. Se han comunicado lesiones renales y hepáticas correspondientes a exposiciones subanestésicas, prolongadas o repetidas a corto plazo. La evaluación de los estudios epidemiológicos se vio dificultada por el pequeño tamaño de las cohortes, la coexposición a cloruro de vinilo y la insuficiente atención al hábito de fumar. Aunque no se encontró una incidencia mayor en grado estadísticamente significativo del cáncer en el hombre expuesto al cloruro de vinilideno, los estudios epidemiológicos fueron insuficientes y no se puede concluir que no entrañe un riesgo carcinogénico. No se dispone de información sobre los efectos del cloruro de vinilideno en la reproducción humana.

2. Evaluación de los efectos en el medio ambiente y riesgos para la salud humana

2.1. Evaluación de los efectos en el medio ambiente

A consecuencia de la volatilización, la atmósfera constituye el principal compartimento ambiental del cloruro de vinilideno. Puesto que la semivida de este compuesto en la troposfera es de unos dos días aproximadamente, parece poco probable que el cloruro de vinilideno contribuya a agotar la capa de ozono de la estratosfera. La lixiviación y la volatilización hacen que el suelo y los sedimentos sean compartimentos ambientales de menor importancia para el cloruro de vinilideno; el nivel de este hidrocarburo clorado en el medio acuoso se ve también reducido al mínimo por la rápida volatilización. No se sabe si la degradación de compuestos como el tricloroetileno y el percloroetileno, que a menudo se encuentran en el agua, contribuye a aumentar apreciablemente los niveles de cloruro de vinilideno en el medio ambiente.

Las concentraciones de cloruro de vinilideno que se observan en las colecciones naturales de agua y los niveles de toxicidad aguda para peces y Daphnia indican que los riesgos de toxicidad aguda para el medio acuático son mínimos. No se dispone de suficientes datos sobre toxicidad a largo plazo para evaluar los efectos subletales sobre los organismos acuáticos que viven en las proximidades de fuentes importantes de contaminación por cloruro de vinilideno, como aguas subterráneas contaminadas y puntos de vertido municipal e industrial.

2.2. Evaluación de los riesgos para la salud humana

2.2.1 Niveles de exposición

La población general está expuesta a niveles muy bajos de cloruro de vinilideno. El nivel máximo notificado en el agua de bebida es de 20 µg/litro, si bien se ha calculado que, en los Estados Unidos de América, la exposición individual diaria del ciudadano medio a través del agua de bebida es de $<0,01$ µg. Los niveles de cloruro de vinilideno en los alimentos no suelen ser detectables; no se han notificado niveles superiores a 10 µg/kg. Los niveles en alimentos derivados de organismos acuáticos se desconocen, pero es probable que sean insignificantes (sección 10.1). Se han comunicado niveles de cloruro de vinilideno en el aire de hasta 52 $\mu g/m^3$ (en el perímetro de una zona industrial). En los Estados Unidos se han comunicado valores medios de concentración en el aire urbano de 20 ng/m^3 en zonas no industriales y 8,7 $\mu g/m^3$ en zonas industriales.

La exposición profesional tiene lugar especialmente en los procesos de producción y polimerización. La respiración es la vía principal de entrada en el organismo y los límites de exposición máximos recomendados o promedios regulados a lo largo de un día de trabajo varían entre 8 y 500 mg/m^3 (o la concentración más baja detectable con un margen de confianza), según el país. Los límites de exposición a corto plazo varían entre 16 y 80 mg/m^3 y los valores máximos entre 50 y 700 mg/m^3. Se ha encontrado que los niveles de cloruro de vinilideno en las atmósferas cerradas a las que algunos trabajadores se ven expuestos no superan los 8 mg/m^3.

2.2.2 Efectos agudos

En el ser humano, es probable que la inhalación de concentraciones elevadas de cloruro de vinilideno (muy aproximadamente iguales o superiores al umbral olfativo máximo de 4000 mg/m^3) provoque depresión del sistema nervioso central y pueda llevar al coma. Basándose en la toxicidad aguda para animales, el cloruro de vinilideno puede ejercer efectos tóxicos en el hígado, el riñón o el pulmón a concentraciones muy inferiores al umbral olfativo mínimo de aproximadamente 2000 mg/m^3. La exposición al cloruro de vinilideno puede producir irritación en los ojos, el tracto respiratorio superior (a 100 mg/m^3 en el hombre, Rylova 1953) y la piel, lo cual se ha atribuido en parte a un agente estabilizante, el p-metoxifenol.

En el ratón, más sensible que la rata a los efectos hapatotóxicos y nefrotóxicos del cloruro de vinilideno, se indujeron lesiones renales por exposición a cantidades tan reducidas como 40 mg de cloruro de vinilideno/m^3 (10 ppm) durante 6 h. También se observaron hepatotoxicidad y nefrotoxicidad notables en la rata. Tras el ayuno, que aumenta la toxicidad, la exposición de la rata a concentraciones de cloruro de vinilideno de 600 mg/m^3 (150 ppm) y 800 mg/m^3 (200 ppm) durante 6 h provocó toxicidad en el hígado y el riñón, respectivamente. Los estudios realizados en la rata indican que la ingestión de alcohol antes de la exposición puede acelerar el metabolismo y exacerbar la toxicidad del cloruro de vinilideno. La toxicidad aguda depende de la especie, el sexo, la estirpe y el régimen de alimentación de los animales. La distinta sensibilidad del ratón y la rata guarda relación con la diferente actividad del metabolismo oxidativo del cloruro de vinilideno en una y otra especie. Aunque no se puede predecir si la rata o el ratón constituyen el modelo más adecuado para el ser humano, la actividad del metabolismo microsómico hepático del hombre es cuantitativamente semejante al de la rata, cuya susceptibilidad es relativamente baja. No hay pruebas de que existan diferencias cualitativas en el metabolismo oxidativo del cloruro de vinilideno en el ser humano y el roedor.

Está claro que el margen entre las concentraciones capaces de producir toxicidad en animales (40 mg/m^3 en el ratón) y los límites de exposición profesional establecidos por algunos países es insuficiente o inexistente.

?.2.3 Efectos a largo plazo y genotoxicidad

La exposición prolongada o repetida a corto plazo a dosis subanestésicas puede producir lesiones renales y hepáticas. Basándose en estudios a largo plazo realizados en animales, en condiciones que simulaban la exposición profesional, se comunicó la aparición de cambios hepáticos a un nivel de exposición de 300 mg/m^3 (75 ppm) en la rata. En el ratón, se observaron lesiones en el riñón y el hígado con 100 mg/m^3 (25 ppm) y 200 mg/m^3 (50 ppm), respectivamente. Los datos sobre sensibilidad a los efectos tóxicos varían considerablemente de unos estudios a otros.

En los animales, el cloruro de vinilideno no parece influir en la capacidad reproductiva ni constituir un riesgo embriotóxico o teratogénico a dosis inferiores a las que producen toxicidad materna, pero este extremo no se ha estudiado en el hombre. Cuando se utilizaron concentraciones capaces de producir toxicidad materna se observaron toxicidad embrionaria y fetal y anomalías fetales, reflejadas en la menor velocidad de aumento de peso.

El cloruro de vinilideno tiene efecto mutagénico en las bacterias y las levaduras siempre que actúe en presencia de un sistema metabólico de mamíferos. También algunas células de mamíferos pueden sufrir lesiones del ADN y efectos mutagénicos in vitro. En la mayoría de los estudios realizados en roedores in vivo no se observaron efectos genotóxicos medidos por la letalidad dominante ni desde el punto de vista citogenético, pero se ha comunicado la observación de aberraciones en células de la médula ósea del hámster chino. El enlace al ADN y la reparación de éste in vivo en roedores fueron detectables pero mínimos. Así pues, los estudios genéticos in vivo sugieren algunos signos de toxicidad genética, pero, en la mayoría de los casos, los efectos fueron mínimos o negativos.

Se han llevado a cabo varios ensayos de carcinogenicidad en tres especies de animales de experimentación (ratones, ratas y hámsters) utilizando diversas vías de administración. Lamentablemente, la mayoría de estos estudios adolecían de graves limitaciones de diseño o de método para la evaluación de la carcinogenicidad. Por vía oral no se observaron efectos carcinogénicos significativos en la rata. En la rata adulta expuesta por inhalación, se notificó un aumento de los tumores de la mama que no guardaba relación con la dosis. Se observó un ligero aumento de la leucemia en las ratas expuestas tanto in utero como recién nacidas. Estas observaciones no pudieron evaluarse. En un estudio realizado en el ratón, se observó una mayor incidencia de adenocarcinomas de riñón en los machos con niveles de exposición de 200 y 100 mg/m^3 (50 y 25 ppm) pero no con 40 y 0 mg/m^3 (10 y 0 ppm). En el mismo estudio, se observaron incidencias estadísticamente mayores de tumores del pulmón (principalmente adenomas en ambos sexos) y carcinomas mamarios (en hembras), pero no se descubrieron relaciones entre la dosis y la respuesta.

Los tumores del riñón pueden estar relacionados de algún modo con la citotoxicidad renal observada; puede ser que las lesiones repetidas del riñón lleven directamente a la respuesta carcinogénica por medio de un mecanismo no genotóxico o bien que faciliten la expresión del potencial genotóxico de los metabolitos en esta especie, este sexo y este órgano en particular. No obstante, esta conclusión es dudosa en la ausencia de datos de dosis-respuesta suficientes sobre los efectos genéticos in vivo, así como ante el descubrimiento de que el cloruro de vinilideno puede haber actuado como iniciador en un ensayo cutáneo en dos etapas en el ratón.

Los estudios epidemiológicos, aunque no dan pruebas estadísticamente significativas de que la exposición profesional al cloruro de vinilideno entrañe un riesgo mayor de cáncer no son adecuados para evaluar debidamente el riesgo carcinogénico del cloruro de vinilideno para el ser humano.

Aunque en las evaluaciones de algunos autores el exceso de defunciones por cáncer se atribuye al azar (a causa del reducido número de sujetos y del tamaño de las cohortes), el hecho de que aparezcan repetidamente valores más altos de lo esperado es digno de mención. En los dos estudios de cohortes comunicados, se observó cáncer del pulmón en 7 casos, cuando cabía esperar 3,16 defunciones. El resultado no puede desecharse, aunque hay que tener presente la coexistencia de la exposición al cloruro de vinilideno (en uno de los estudios). Puesto que las cohortes se determinaron según su exposición al cloruro de vinilideno, puede ser imposible excluir otras exposiciones que induzcan a error. Las conclusiones comunicadas en materia de morbilidad (incluido un caso de carcinoma testicular) pueden ser útiles a título informativo. La interpretación por parte de los autores de que la mayor morbilidad hepática guardaba relación con el consumo de alcohol por los sujetos no es válida, puesto que no se evaluó la ingestión de alcohol por todos los sujetos del estudio (y no sólo por los casos identificados).

3. Recomendaciones

3.1 Recomendaciones para trabajos futuros

Es preciso disponer de mejores estimaciones de la producción mundial anual de cloruro de vinilideno y de las cantidades de cloruro de vinilideno que ingresan en el medio ambiente de todas las procedencias, ya sea en forma de cloruro de vinilideno como tal o por la degradación de otros productos químicos.

El destino ambiental previsto se basa en escasas pruebas experimentales. Se necesita más información sobre las tasas de degradación y sobre los productos de transformación en el aire, el suelo, el agua y los sedimentos, y el metabolismo en especies no mamíferas representativas.

Deben llevarse a cabo estudios de toxicidad a largo plazo en los que se investiguen los diversos punto finales patológicos en especies acuáticas representativas (peces, crustáceos y moluscos). Deben definirse con más precisión los umbrales y los mecanismos de los efectos tóxicos que tiene la exposición al cloruro de vinilideno a corto y a largo plazo en el animal y el ser humano, como base para establecer niveles seguros de exposición.

Conviene hacer un uso más exhaustivo de los datos existentes en materia de carcinogenicidad. Los nuevos estudios sobre carcinogenicidad deben hacerse según un protocolo aceptado de bioensayo durante un lapso de vida entera que tenga en cuenta específicamente las propiedades particulares del cloruro de vinilideno. Esos estudios deben tener presentes la brevedad de la semivida de la sustancia en el organismo, la importancia de la edad al comienzo de la exposición, la duración de la exposición diaria y otros datos pertinentes que puedan estar relacionados con el establecimiento del régimen de dosificación. Hay que seleccionar cuidadosamente las especies y estirpes de los animales de experimentación. Los datos de toxicidad así como los datos metabólicos y farmacocinéticos correspondientes a estos animales también serían sumamente útiles.

Deben llevarse a cabo estudios de seguimiento a largo plazo sobre la morbilidad y la mortalidad en poblaciones enteras y no seleccionadas expuestas al cloruro de vinilideno.

Se necesitan estudios epidemiológicos que permitan evaluar los efectos de la exposición al cloruro de vinilideno (incluida la exposición prolongada a niveles reducidos) en poblaciones humanas. Es particularmente necesario disponer de información sobre efectos como la aparición precoz de enfermedades cerebrovasculares y cáncer; los estudios deben tener en cuenta los factores que introducen errores, como el hábito de fumar y el consumo de alcohol (posiblemente en un sistema de referencia de casos).

Debe recurrirse a datos históricos como base de comparación con los resultados de las investigaciones en curso para poder evaluar los efectos protectores que han tenido las medidas de reglamentación durante los últimos años.

Para las investigaciones tanto en curso como futuras, un medio valioso de salvar el problema del reducido número de sujetos que hay en cada lugar de producción por separado sería aunar todos los datos de éstos y realizar estudios multicéntricos. Debe investigarse en animales de experimentación el valor de la utilización de un agente con grupo sulfhidrilo como la N-acetilcisteína en el tratamiento de la intoxicación por cloruro de vinilideno.

Es necesario comparar la farmacocinética y el metabolismo in vivo/in vitro del cloruro de vinilideno, especialmente en el riñón, el hígado y el pulmón, en animales de experimentación de distintas especies y en el ser humano, con el fin de comprender mejor los resultados obtenidos en estudios de toxicidad in vivo. Se precisan datos paralelos sobre la genotoxicidad potencial del cloruro de vinilideno en el lugar escogido para estudiar la carcinogénesis en distintas especies a fin de examinar el posible papel de un mecanismo genético.

A la luz de las conclusiones neurotoxicológicas comunicadas en el presente análisis, es necesario investigar el papel de los sistemas moduladores en la patogénesis de la intoxicación por cloruro de vinilideno.

3.2 Protección personal y tratamiento de la intoxicación

3.2.1 Protección personal

En los lugares de trabajo en la industria donde pueden producirse exposiciones a corto plazo por inhalación superiores a los límites recomendados, deben utilizarse mascarillas faciales completas con filtro para los vapores orgánicos y, en previsión de una emergencia, deben proporcionarse mascarillas con sistema de abastecimiento de aire. Para evitar el contacto con el cuerpo, los operarios que manejen cloruro de vinilideno deben llevar ropa protectora, en buen estado, que incluya gafas de seguridad. Debe mantenerse una ventilación constante dentro de las plantas industriales mediante respiraderos con filtros en los lugares donde puedan producirse derrames o fugas. Se recomienda vigilar las emisiones de cloruro de vinilideno durante las operaciones de distribución. En caso de una fuga, debe forzarse la evaporación del cloruro de vinilideno ya sea directamente si se trata de una cantidad pequeña o por evaporación controlada utilizando una espuma sintética de expansión. Para disperar los vapores de la espuma pueden utilizarse aspersores de agua en cortinas.

3.2.2 Tratamiento de la intoxicación en el hombre

En casos de exposición excesiva o de ingestión, debe consultarse a un médico. Dadas las propiedades irritantes del cloruro de vinilideno, debe prestarse especial atención a los pulmones, la piel y los ojos. Deben vigilarse las funciones del corazón, el hígado, el riñón y el sistema nervioso central. Puesto que los datos correspondientes a animales indican que el cloruro de vinilideno produce un aumento notable de la sensibilidad a las arritmias cardiacas inducidas por la adrenalina, debe evitarse el empleo de este fármaco. La hipotensión grave puede tratarse por transfusión, con sangre entera o sustitutos del plasma. No se conoce antídoto alguno.

Un paciente intoxicado por inhalación de cloruro de vinilideno debe mantenerse abrigado en posición semiprona y en una atmósfera bien ventilada y fresca. Las vías respiratorias deben mantenerse despejadas y debe administrarse oxígeno si el sujeto se encuentra en estado de estupor o de coma. En caso necesario debe aplicarse respiración artificial.

Tras la ingestión de cloruro de vinilideno debe enjuagarse la boca con agua. No debe provocarse el vómito por el riesgo de aspiración de cloruro de vinilideno hacia la laringe y los pulmones. El lavado gástrico y/o la administración oral de carbono activado o de parafina líquida pueden ayudar a reducir la biodisponibilidad de cloruro de vinilideno si se administran dentro de la hora que sigue a la ingestión, pero pueden beneficiar al paciente hasta 4 horas después de la ingestión.

Los ojos expuestos a cloruro de vinilideno deben irrigarse inmediatamente con agua durante más de 15 minutos y debe acudirse al médico.

En caso de exposición cutánea, las ropas contaminadas deben retirarse y debe lavarse la zona afectada con agua y jabón.

www.ingramcontent.com/pod-product-compliance
Ingram Content Group UK Ltd.
Pitfield, Milton Keynes, MK11 3LW, UK
UKHW021312180426
11947UKWH00015B/1172